I WANT TO SLEEP

UNLEARNING INSOMNIA
TREAT YOURSELF TO A GOOD NIGHT

Siegfried F. Haug

SIEGFRIED HAUG

Outskirts Press, Inc.
Denver, Colorado

Outskirts Press, Inc.
http://www.outskirtspress.com

ISBN: 978-1-4327-2072-8

Library of Congress Control Number: 2008927113

Outskirts Press and the "OP" logo are trademarks belonging to Outskirts Press, Inc.

PRINTED IN THE UNITED STATES OF AMERICA

To my father:

He always asked how the book was coming.

ACKNOWLEDGMENTS

I want to thank the people who made this book possible.

Jane Hillman for supporting me throughout the arduous process. There were many times when you had more confidence in me and the book than I did and your suggestions made it more readable.

Sue Freeman, for such patient reading and advising. You worked your way through not only one, but three drafts of this book. I appreciate your diligence, your gentleness, and your skill.

Ellie Cook, for professional copyediting.
What a relief to have you on my side.

Carol Hillman for having faith and plying me with writerly support.

Thank you, Evan Daniels, Joel Spiro and Leigh Bailey, Frank Demaree, Jeff Farrell, Bruno Buissière, and Premila Nair for being readers.

Thanks, also, to the many people who asked for my professional help and provided me with motivation, material, and the vision to begin and finish writing.

Then, I want to acknowledge the staff of Outskirts Press. Especially Elizabeth Javor for her responsiveness. Writing a book is one thing, getting someone to publish it quite another.

For all this collective effort I am grateful.

TABLE OF CONTENTS

FOREWORD

Some time ago I spent an overnight in a hospital. Although I shared a room with another woman, the curtain between our beds prevented any glimpse of or interaction with her. What I knew about her came from snippets of overheard conversation that revealed her consternation over unremitting back pain despite the procedure that she had just endured. Most relevant for me, however, was the fact that this was night, and her sleep behavior did not remotely match mine. From what I could gather, her television was on and stayed on all night long. It was not so much the sound that hindered my attempt to sleep, but rather the light that a television commonly emits. I am fairly certain that most people know that a flickering television light precludes and interrupts the deepest sleep, and I was sure that my roommate craved unconsciousness as much, if not more than I did. However, I know too that people often are aware of 'what is good for them,' but do otherwise.

I am aware that many people have televisions in their bedrooms and watch them as part of their bedtime ritual; they even can be set to turn off automatically in the event that the viewer has fallen asleep. I am not one of those people. I have a different bedtime ritual, one that is fairly methodical and seems to work for me. It does not include a television but rather some quiet reflection and reading just before lights out. I trust that there are other ways for people to end their wakefulness, and I have frequently asked my clients what they do to 'wind down' at bedtime. Many have not discovered a reliable path to sleep. This book that represents the cumulative wisdom and experience of Dr. Haug in conjunction with his patients' journeys, contributes significantly to helping people consistently find their path to sleep.

As a practicing psychologist, I have heard about sleep difficulties just as Dr. Haug has. Friends, too, have expressed their own trials and tribulations in relation to sleep. In some cases these lapses can readily be attributed to a temporary crisis, troubling or traumatic life event. Even after this passes or is resolved, sleep can remain elusive. Physicians may tell patients that they have broken the 'sleep habit,' and a brief stint of medication will get them back on track. The medication may work so well that people become reluctant to relinquish it. If and when they do their anxiety about sleep comes to the fore. As Dr. Haug documents, not sleeping is a fearsome prospect. To avoid anxiety at the prospect of wakefulness, people will continue the medication or try using television as a lullaby. These remedies are called iatrogenic when the cure becomes more formidable than the original symptom it was used to alleviate. People now need to cure both their dependency on medications and their sleep difficulties.

Dr. Haug astutely addresses these complications in stories from his practice. Why another book on sleep? Much is known about sleep and what brings it about. Findings from research studies and sleep centers are frequently published in popular press venues. The steps needed to sleep are finite and fairly simple. Knowing what to do, however, is a far cry from actually doing it. Dr. Haug's cases clearly demonstrate the complications that deter people from changing their patterns even when desperate for sleep. To witness these stories enables readers to feel compassion for themselves and to identify with others engaged in a common struggle. What seems so simple, sleep, is not. We have obscured our path to sleep and need help and encouragement to find our way back to this basic and critical human need. A lack of sleep increases our vulnerability to physical and emotional distress. We cannot wait for sleep to come to us, in the form of a childlike 'sandman.'

Dr. Haug shows us instead that we must 'go to sleep,' embrace sleep and allow it to replenish and heal us daily. In education we emphasize stories as effective instruction. Here Dr. Haug uses stories to teach us, to provide examples where readers may find some aspects of themselves or their experience, and to supply information about sleep behavior and its antithesis. These stories attest to the difficulty of finding our way back to our primary need for sleep. Ultimately, they give clarity and hope to allow us to literally "go to sleep."

Sue J. M. Freeman, Ph.D.
Licensed Psychologist
Professor, Smith College
Northampton, Massachusetts

PROLOGUE

O sleep! O gentle sleep!
Nature's soft nurse,
How have I frightened thee
That thou no more
Wilt weigh my eyelids down
And steep my senses
In forgetfulness?

William Shakespeare,
Henry IV, Part 2

I hear you are writing a book on insomnia.

We are sitting on the couch together, catching up.

Well, I say, *not really.*

So many people, I find, want to talk about insomnia. Relatives, friends, colleagues, strangers on the plane; It is amazing how many people don't get the sleep they want.

The book, I try to explain, *is about getting the sleep you want.*

Okay, he smiles indulgently as if I had been mincing words, *how do I get the sleep I want, then?*

By putting your mind at ease, I say.

Just like that. He sounds a trifle sarcastic so I don't say anything.

There's gotta be more to it than that, he says.

No, I say, *that's about it.*

All I need to do is set my mind at ease and I'll get to sleep?

More likely than not, I say.

I see, he says, *the trick is to get your mind to be at ease because when you are an insomniac it obviously isn't.*

Yep, I say, *that's the trick.*

And, ah ... how do you do that?

You start by not doing the things that make your mind uneasy. I say.

Like what?

Like scaring yourself.

He looks confused.

Look, I say, *if I give you a hundred bucks to keep yourself from sleeping tonight would you know how to do it?*

2

I WANT TO SLEEP

I never thought about it, he says, *but yeah, I guess I could do that.*

So you know how to keep yourself awake?

Yes, drink lots of coffee, call people, worry about my taxes, get pissed at my ex, wonder about what my kids are up to. I could do it.

Excellent, I say. *You already know how to work with your mind, then. Now if I gave you a hundred bucks to get a good night's sleep—would you know how to make that happen?*

Without drugs?

Without drugs, I say.

He hesitates.

Well, I say, *that's what the book is about. If you can do one thing to your mind, like agitating it, maybe there is a way you can give it a rest.*

If you really wanted, that is.

INTRODUCTION

Millions of people worldwide can't sleep. Insomnia has reached epidemic proportions, and short of knocking yourself out chemically, there seem to be few reliable methods to coax a mind into sleep-mode.

New medications are being developed at a rapid pace, and sleep clinics offer their services in any major town. Medications though have side-effects and sleep clinics mainly target sleep apnea.

What about plain insomnia? I asked the director of a local sleep center.

Well, he said, *these are the people we don't quite know what to do with.*

Why is that? I wanted to know.

Because most of their problems are psychological, he said.

"Psychological" is a word doctors use when a complaint doesn't have a clear physiological or biological explanation, which means there is no likely pharmacological treatment.

It's in your head, many of us were told; the implication being that the pain was somehow less than real.

You are making it up; get over it!

The people who come to see me know by and large that their sleep problems are in their head. They also know it is not that simple. After all: love, hope, faith, fear, and grief are in your head too. A lot of fear. Others, who are convinced that a biological etiology to their disease is all there is to it, don't seek counseling.

So much, I believe, is clear to most who are sleep-challenged: One part of you wants to sleep; another part— in your mind—obstructs it. It usually does so by making it look as if wide-awake worrying was necessary, legitimate, "good," and un-avoidable. In effect it does so by scaring you.

That is not necessary and it certainly is not good. But first you'll have to distinguish and appreciate the difference between "being scared" and "scaring yourself." They are not the same. One causes the other.

Knowing that difference can help you change what is happening in your mind. Running scary scenarios in your mind is a widely accepted motivational tool to kick you into high gear performance-wise. It is obviously deadly for sleep purposes.

A wired mind puts you on high alert. A tired mind prepares for sleep by letting your guard down.

Those two purposes or mind-sets pull in different

directions. At night, just as you want to go to sleep, this internal conflict comes to a head. The result is what we call *insomnia*. Insomnia is a form of internal war and—like in all wars—everybody loses in the end. One could almost say insomnia wars are territorial because "wired" and "tired" parts of us compete for the same space at the same time.

This is a non scientific, quasi-poetic way of addressing a neurological process called the 'sleep-switch'. Researchers at Harvard Medical School have isolated a neural struggle for dominance in our brain. Neuromodulators from the front of the hypothalamus compete with opposing 'forces' from the posterior lateral hypothalamus. The former activate sleep while the latter keep us awake. If you don't want to lose the battle to the posterior laterals, you need to do something about it. Drugs, of course, would be one thing. Short of that you'd need to learn how to intervene in your own behalf. You need to make your preference known, because the wired way of life is dominant from picking up momentum all day long. When you consciously intercede, your thinking steps in-between the two. The two of them—"wired", and "tired"—become separate, distinguished, as you give yourself pause. Time enough to take sides. At night, for NOW you want to side with the tired part of you.

That means letting go, temporarily turning your back on the wired part, which is both scared and scary.

The ensuing process is one of mending the oppositional relationship you have with yourself.

As you intervene in the relationship between those two— the part that is tired and wants to sleep, and the part that is wired and needs to stay awake—you do basic self-care.

As you do basic self-care you are once again on the same page with sleep, because this is what sleep does best: It takes care of you in the most effective way known to humankind.

This book is about what's going on in your head when you want to sleep and your mind won't let you. It is about listening to it, assessing it, and changing it.

We are now led to believe insomnia is a curse and instructed to act accordingly.

What if it is a blessing? Disguised, for sure, like most of them? An invitation, maybe, to make lifestyle changes that serve us better?

WHAT YOU WILL FIND

What you'll find in the pages ahead are stories of people not unlike you who had trouble sleeping. Gradually, in processes lasting from weeks to months, they unlearned their insomnia. That means they decided against being a scary, impatient presence and learned how to be comforting and soothing to themselves instead. There are many other ways to say the same thing. It means that they turned from fighting insomnia to enabling sleep. Instead of catering to the wired part in themselves, they embraced the tired. On a basic level they started spending time on/with themselves, patiently.

At times, that translated into nightly episodes of catching up, listening, and soothing. At times it required reclaiming days and nights from schedules that would scare anybody's sleep away. In the end their search for sleep yielded much more than what they thought they had lost. It turned out they hadn't just lost sleep; they were in the process of losing their way, their place, and their sense of worth. Their lives were driven by stimuli rather than values, and they were in danger of selling out to a world where peace of mind is for losers, and sleep is a waste of time. In relationship terms, they had grown apart inside, and it was insomnia that prompted a reconciliation.

These case stories are followed by wrap-up commentaries; attempts to put the processes larger contexts.

At this stage this is just talk. Walking the walk, however, involves many, sometimes inconsequential-looking steps. Some of those steps literally seem pedestrian when you look at them out of context. Nevertheless, I have provided a *Basics* list for you in the following chapter. This list of basics is further detailed in the *workbook* component of this book. To watch those fundamental tools at work, immerse yourself in the stories and see if you can recognize yourself in some of them.

BASICS

Sleep is not a performance or a commodity. It is a gift to those who are willing to surrender control. *Basically you want to learn how to switch your presence, your allegiance, from the wired to the tired parts in your mind.*

You are no longer charged to make things happen. You are getting ready to present yourself to sleep so IT can take over. Attitudinally speaking, you become patient and present. It is now sleeping-time. Sleep can't be rushed. Behaviorally, that translates into a switch from scaring yourself to soothing yourself.

Think of being present as turning to face a person and maybe even offering a smile and an embrace. There is a German word for that: *Zuwendung.* Turning and becoming present, including to yourself, has basic attitudinal features and behavioral requirements. Just as not-being-present has.

Being *not* present is an upsetting experience for everyone involved, and this is how it's done:

- You don't listen.
- You don't care.
- You are unavailable.
- You are disruptive.

- You are dismissive and belittling.
- You create distance.
- You are impatient.

When you switch to being present it is foremost a gift of *time*.

- You give yourself the time of day or night.
- You start paying attention.
- You listen with empathy.
- You stay focused.
- You put your own 'stuff' on hold for the time being.
- You are soothing and comforting.
- You validate.
- Your closeness invites confidences.

In the stories that make up the body of this book, you'll see these principles at work. You'll witness people not being present to themselves, and maybe you can even watch the *Zuwendung* happen as they get to be better sleepers over time. Once you get into the spirit of those journeys you might be able to relate to whatever it is you need at that time.

Insomnia forces and affords an encounter with yourself. Changing it from a scary, negative encounter to a soothing one is what this book advocates and teaches.

In the appendix you will find a detailed listing of basic techniques and how to put them to use. Techniques are generally overrated because, like tools, they are only as good as the person who knows how and when to use them.

If you want to use techniques in the spirit of getting things done *faster*, you are on the wrong track. The spirit of sleeping comes in the form of patience. Insomnia makes you come face to face with your rushed and rushing self.

For now, though, forget about techniques and let yourself enter the stories.

CHAPTER 1
I CAN'T FALL ASLEEP

Bed is a medicine.

Italian proverb

F or a highly functioning person, going to sleep often becomes a control issue. Most people with insomnia wish they could control their sleep onset, and usually try to do so by every means possible. When that fails their anxiety level goes up, and sleep retreats even further. Eventually they become terrified of losing one more nightly battle and dread going to bed. Their nightly alone time has become a battlefield. Medication looks like a way to reestablish some control until dependency makes a mockery of it.

CHERYL

Cheryl found me on the Internet. My name had come up as part of the *Psychology Today* network, specialty: insomnia. She hadn't slept in months, as she told me over the phone. Not without Ambien anyway.

I wouldn't know what to do without it, she said, expressing a sentiment that I have heard a lot over the past years.

At our first appointment Cheryl confessed to some guilt and uneasiness. Her regular therapist, a psychologist in a neighboring town, had advised her against consulting with an insomnia specialist.

You are already totally obsessed with your sleep problems, he told her. *The last thing you need is to talk about it some more.*

She respected her therapist greatly as he had helped her through a difficult year with breast cancer but felt that she needed to do something *drastic* about her fear of going to bed.

I agreed that obsessing was probably a bad idea, especially at two o'clock in the morning with nothing to disrupt the process.

She laughed. *If I could stop obsessing, I probably would be halfway there sleeping-wise.*

To myself I thought: *Not halfway, Cheryl, all the way.*

Had she done anything about her "brain that wouldn't quit"?

Well, yes, her therapist had recommended Zoloft, an antidepressant also known for its effectiveness with obsessive ruminations and some compulsive behaviors. She hadn't been on it that long (two months) but thought it might be working—some.

Do you know when you are obsessing? I asked.

No, she laughed, *but my co-workers do. They tell me all the time to stop obsessing.* Then, serious again, *but then they don't have to report to the board.*

Well, I said, *maybe if you caught yourself obsessing you could do something about it.*

I am certainly obsessing at night, she said, *no difficulty catching THAT. And recently I have started obsessing about getting into bed, knowing I'd obsess.*

Then that would be the perfect place to start, I smiled: *For you to know that you have a problem with obsessing and not necessarily with sleep is a tremendous insight.*

I usually spend a good part of the first appointment finding out as much as possible what specifically got a person to spend time and money to see me. With sleep-deprived people, however, I have relaxed that rule. They are desperate for a tool, a mere hint, a trick, even, that might make the coming night a less terrifying experience.

Cheryl did not quite know what to do with me complimenting her about her 'tremendous insight'.

I don't see the difference between obsessing and not being able to sleep. Aren't they the same?

No, they are as different as cause and effect, I said, *you can't make yourself sleep but you can get off an obsessive merry-go-round.*

I can? How?

Magic, I said, *the ancient magic of gaining power by knowing your adversary's name.*

Many cultures retain an awareness that knowing a name is power. For that reason indigenous people often have a secret name that only close allies know. The right words will open the vital door. Or close it. Knowing its name will compel the genie to become your servant.

Magical power. Word power; disguise-lifting power.

Tonight, Cheryl, when you catch yourself obsessing, say: "Cheryl, you are obsessing."

And that'll stop it?

It will interrupt it. Like interrupting someone who is on a rampage. You are inserting a space, a pause. Into that space you can then insert something else. Something better.

Like what?

Like five minutes' worth of intentional breathing; like some gentle unkinking of stiff muscles—or even more effectively—by telling yourself a story that makes you smile and soothes the soul.

That makes sense, Cheryl said, *I'll try that.*

It will be a start, I said. *But there is more.*
Ask your friends at work how they can tell when you are getting white-knuckled about something.

She looked puzzled.

I WANT TO SLEEP

There are physical changes when a person gets caught up in an obsessive state of mind, I said. *The face looks different, breathing changes, voice quality, diction, and demeanor...they all get altered.*

Cheryl looked a bit lost.

You are wondering how that relates to sleep?

I know that it relates to sleep –somehow, she said. *What I don't know is what to do about it.*

Intellectual insight is one thing. Making changes is quite another. This clearly had been a sore point in many earlier discussions, therapeutic and otherwise.

What do your co-workers do when they call you on your obsessing?

They laugh and, well, call me on it.

Then what?

Then I snap out of it for a while—sometimes.

The magic of calling it by name, I said.

Woman, thy name is obsession, Cheryl smiled.

Are you ready for some serious homework? I asked.

She went for her spiral notebook.

One: keep minutes. Take some time right after our session

and record everything you remember that might have relevance for your quest. What is your quest, by the way?

Conquer insomnia, she said determinedly.

May I suggest a rewording? How about paving the way for sleep?

Isn't that six of one and a half dozen of the other?

No, I said. *Conquering insomnia is just another obsession, a nightly fight. Embracing sleep is a peacemaking mission. Different spirit.*

She wrote it down.

Two? she said.

Two is getting the identifying data for what Cheryl looks like when she obsesses.

From my co-workers?

Yes. Three: Pick four visual/bodily features they point out like: "your jaw gets all set"; or "you stare ahead without blinking and barely breathing" or "you start fidgeting."

Tapping my finger, she smiled; *pinching my lips.* She demonstrated.

Four: at home in front of a mirror, do those things.

Pretend? she said.

I WANT TO SLEEP

Method acting, I said and she smiled.

Acting the bitch, she said, *shouldn't be too hard.*

For one minute: frown, tap pinch. Then do some breathing. Another round of looking obsessed and uptight. Then breathe.

Five: Tonight lie in wait for the obsessive act to start.

Six: Say its name. Break the curse, as you have practiced, and watch it wither.

Seven, she said, *CUT.*

You got it, I said.

This shift from frantically fighting insomnia to doing things sleep likes is crucial if you want to have restorative nights again. You can't force sleep to come to you—you can, however, work your way back to where sleep is waiting for you. Sleep is waiting for you but not where the wild goose chases take place.

Sleep is our birthright. Short of serious mental or medical conditions our whole being is set up for sleeping. Sleep is not the problem—being awake is. On a certain level sleep is always there; ready to take us on like stepping back into an ancient river. But during the day we scramble for the hills that seem to hold all promise. Our craving for excitement, our agitated minds run away from sleep. All day long we push ourselves in the opposite direction from where sleep resides –until we decide it is time for going unconscious. Then we want sleep to come (to us.) Then and there, when sleep isn't where we want it to be, we call it insomnia, and feel betrayed and even more worried when sleep isn't where we think it should be. Sleep can't follow us into wired wide-wake country. We need to go back to where sleep lives.

By the time people come to me they have tried everything that Internet searches could yield: special teas, acupressure points, Chinese herbs, homeopathic remedies, vitamins, and minerals. These cures oftentimes have positive results, sometimes for extended periods of time; then, for some people the insomnia-fighting powers of their 'helpers' become unreliable and wane.

I believe this is because insomnia-fighting in itself is a counterproductive paradigm. All manner of fighting is counter to sleep readiness.

Sleep on demand is not what it is all about.

Sleep requires peace of mind, and the happy relief it brings. Peace in the bedroom, peace in the digestive tract, peace in your hormonal output, peace in your last e-mail.

The more peace, the safer our organism feels. Unsafe organisms stay vigilant. Feeling safe, MAKING safe is the emotional route to sleep.

People get turned off when I make this speech. Workshop participants dutifully try to take notes; readers, I suppose, read it.

I knew Cheryl wanted and desperately hoped for something to DO come bedtime that night. I also knew that she considered learning about her obsessing somewhat of a waste of time, or certainly not something central to her quest. If her quest only could be changed from defeating insomnia to enabling sleep—from staying with the wired to standing by the *tired*. It would head her in the right direction.

Intercepting an obsessive sequence, getting off the subject, letting go of nagging worries is one of the most powerful sleep-enabling skills a person could ever hope to master.

So I said: *In the meantime there are some things you can do. Think of them as tools in an emergency kit. Some you know already. They all will get better if you use them regularly and often.*

Cheryl had her notebook ready.

1. *You need to learn the difference between being scared and scaring yourself.*
2. *You need to learn to become fully awake.*
3. *You need to learn to breathe intentionally for about five minutes at a time.*
4. *You need to learn to unkink your body without risking cramps.*
5. *You need to learn to say comforting words to yourself.*
6. *You need to start telling yourself emotionally pleasing bedtime stories.*

When I conduct a workshop, this list goes on the whiteboard. Hardly ever do I get a question like: *How do you tell a bedtime story to yourself?* Or: *What do you mean—becoming fully awake?*

People take these tools at face value and rarely see anything remarkable about them. As concepts they are indeed easy to get. *I know that, I've done that!* Walking the walk, though, in the middle of the night is another story.

Cheryl, however, looked up: *I don't get the 'wakeup' part. I AM awake.*

You are not awake enough to make the breathing happen. At best you are fitfully resting, which is not restful at all.

You can say that again, Cheryl said. *But I don't see the difference between being scared and scaring myself. Seems like the same thing to me.*

It isn't, I said. *Scaring yourself is what you do before you end up all upset.*

Always? She asked.

No, not always, I said. *Sometimes there are nameless fears in your bones. For now let's deal with scares that come in words.*

On the way out she asked: *One more word of wisdom for the road?*

No coffee, I said.

I don't drink coffee.

What do you drink?

Tea.

I WANT TO SLEEP

What kind?

Green tea, she said; *organic.*

Green tea has caffeine, I said.

It does?

I wasn't sure if she was teasing.

I oftentimes don't suggest a follow-up appointment after the first session just to make sure the person returns on their own accord.

Cheryl called me that day from work: *We didn't set another appointment.*

Did you type up your minutes yet? I said.

Not yet—do I have to have them by next week?

Absolutely, I said.

COMMENTARY

There are many reasons why people can't fall asleep. Obsessive mental processing—*too much on the mind*—is by far the most frequent and effective way to prolong the agony. It is this process that removes people from sleeping as effectively as if they were intentionally running in the opposite direction. So, being able to exit this process is a tremendously valuable step in the right direction. First, of course, you have to catch yourself in the act. Then you need to know what to do instead.

What I hoped to suggest to Cheryl, in this introductory session, was that she might have more control over her sleep-adverse behavior than she thought she had. More say means less victimization. Less victimization means more safety, less fear, and maybe a better chance for sleep.

Session Two

Always the administrator, Cheryl had called the day before to confirm her appointment.

Well, she started, *I actually had some pretty decent nights.*

Job well done, I said. *How did you do it?*

You mean I am not all bad? she said, only half in jest.

You wouldn't be here if you were, I said.

I am not sure I know exactly what I did differently, Cheryl continued, *but I think I went to bed feeling not the same way. Less scared, maybe?*

Mmhm ... How do you think that came about?

She said she no idea. *Maybe it was a less stressful week—even though I can't think why it should have been.*

Cheryl appeared more relaxed and had come thoroughly prepared. Her minutes revealed a take on our last session that—as always—had its unique and unexpected twist.

I WANT TO SLEEP

I hate it when that bitchy side of me comes out. (She was referring to her obsessive interactions with co-workers)

If it didn't come out, I said, *it would stay in, and you might never be able to see it and face up to it—or face it down as the case might be.*

The discussion that followed was significant for the rest of Cheryl's work with me and with herself.

She had, like most of us, used the concept of *being one's own best friend* many times. As a matter of fact she had made the appointment with me because an acquaintance had told her that she owed it to herself and she deserved it. But mostly *being her own best friend* had remained a mere manner of speaking.

Over the next several weeks she encountered the real thing. Watching her internal dialogue, she noticed how she treated herself and talked to herself, and most frighteningly, the low opinion she had of herself. None of that was new or original; after all she had been in therapy for a long time, and owned *yards of self-help books.* She knew about self-loathing and how *bad* it was, about affirmations, and how we should treat ourselves well.

This, however, was different. Sleepless, it dawned on her that the reason for her anxiety, and her dread of yet another night was that she was stuck with herself, feared herself, and did not want to be alone with herself. Being alone with herself without the distracting opportunities of work and social life, TV, telephone, and Blackberry prompts was hell. She knew how to obsess, but not how to be kindly at peace with herself. Looking at insomnia with new eyes brought that home.

I have been working on that stuff for a decade now, and it is getting me depressed she said; *I hate being alone with myself. It's like being in a bad marriage. It could drive a person to drink.*

You have been 'working on it'? I asked.

Yes. I want to like myself.

How do you work on the relationship with your friends?

I go out of my way to do nice things; I am generous to a fault...

So, it's not so much of a feeling, I suggested.

It's mostly what you do, she said.

What stops you from doing loving things for yourself? I asked.

I guess I've been waiting for the feeling to come, you know?

How about trying it the other way around, I said. *Do the nice things and see if the feelings will follow.*

Isn't that kind of fake?

Maybe, I said, *but it sure beats waiting for some feeling to come around. Anyway, how much DO you drink?*

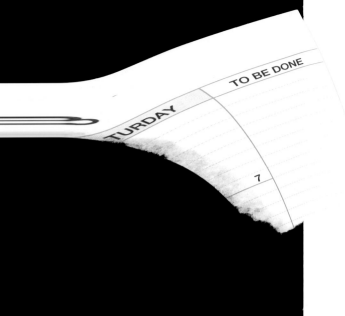

I WANT TO SLEEP

Not as much as I used to and not as much as my sainted brother. Maybe two glasses a night. Not hard stuff—Merlot; Australian.

Too much.

She bristled.

One—I held up a finger—*you shouldn't drink while you are on Zoloft. Two*—*you shouldn't have alcohol while you are nibbling on Ambien. Three*—*alcohol is a diuretic; it truncates your sleep, messes with your dreams, and makes you go to the bathroom when you could be sleeping.*

Two glasses of wine at night is not exactly alcoholism! She was not happy with my list of contraindications.

Plus, I said, undeterred, *alcohol is a depressant; not the mood-elevator you were hoping for.*

Two measly glasses!?

I laughed, and after an attempt at looking put out, she laughed with me.

Homework, I said:

Get yourself a decent sleep book; a blank journal to keep taking notes. Leather-bound. Nothing but the best. You deserve it. Write in it especially when you are in the waiting room for sleep. Imagine corresponding with your best girlfriend. Keep her posted, catch her up. Tell her about your nightly encounters with yourself. Cut back to one glass.

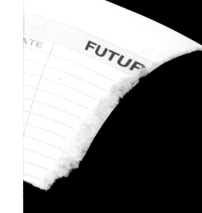

The bottle will go stale.

Let it breathe.

Eat no later than seven if you are turning in by eleven. TV out by ten. Same for the computer.

WHAT?? She moaned.

Switch to decaf teas.

Close your bedroom door on Morris.

He won't like it and meow all night long!

Didn't you tell me that he walks all over you, paws your chest, and nibbles on your ears?

Yes, but ...

Get earplugs.

Anything else? she said prissily, and decisively closed her spiral notebook.

COMMENTARY

Finding your way back to sleep is a lifestyle change. It's little things you DO. Don't wait until you feel like it. Doing these things invokes the spirit of self-care of which sleep is the guardian. There is a constant temptation to bargain and cheat when it comes to modifying routines. After all, they were originally designed for comfort and temporary ease.

However, some things are just not negotiable. That is hard for people who are flexible and expect flexibility.

- Obsessing removes you from sleep no matter how legitimate your concerns.
- Worrying is scary. It might motivate the wired, you but it will betray the tired you.
- Alcohol is bad for sleep continuity. It might initially knock you out, but later it will seriously deteriorate your sleep-patterns. If used as self-medication, night after night, you are running a very real risk of becoming addicted.
- Cats and other pets, or snoring spouses, as we shall see in another chapter, might be comforting initially, but you are guaranteed to be woken up several times during the night. Not a good thing for a light sleeper.
- A big meal in the evening metabolizes into caloric output—energy—when you want and need it least: in the middle of the night.

The devil, therapeutically speaking, is in the details of instituting little changes. It is one thing to embrace the idea of using presleep time as an exclusive rendezvous with yourself. It is quite another to guard it by keeping your cat out.

For the most part, insomnia has become an accepted "cultural signature behavior," a generalized common condition affecting many millions of people, from Australia to Zimbabwe. There is usually not one big traumatic event that causes these sleep problems but rather many little, socially conditioned and even expected habits that finally add up and gain critical, symptomatic mass. Because anti-sleep behaviors are omnipresent, accepted, and automatic, they are hard to catch and tedious to deal with. They grow on you unnoticed, and confronting them might isolate you from your cohorts.

There it is: Sleep doesn't like unsettled minds, excited nervous systems, and raised voices. It does not care about late-breaking news and gossipy relationship disasters.

Going back to sleep means doing things the sleep way.

Session 3

Several weeks passed before I saw Cheryl again. A business trip had taken her to the West Coast, and she decided to stop over in Phoenix and visit her mother.

Part of her catching-up strategy upon returning was to schedule all her overdue appointments within a couple of days. When she saw me that day, she had talked to her "regular shrink"—her term—only hours ago.

I wonder if insomnia isn't really a disease, you know?

Well, I said, *several forms of it are listed in the DSM* (Diagnostic Statistical Manual) *as sleep disorders.*

Do I qualify? she wanted to know.

Yes, you definitely do, I said.

So? Cheryl challenged.

I WANT TO SLEEP

So you can confidently submit my bill to your insurance company. Other than that, a diagnosis does not specify treatment.

Therapists know, and prospective clients might want to know, that therapy, like most relationships, has a honeymoon phase. Then the work starts, and the testing of the person whom you have entrusted with coaching you along a better way.

Insomnia is listed as a genuine disease; YOU say it's a mere symptom, a plea – who is to say ...? She said.

Cheryl had read up on the subject, of that I was sure, and she had returned because something in our talks had made personal sense.

A symptom is a message and a messenger, I said. *It tells you something about yourself you need to know, like running a temp. I don't believe that shooting the messenger is a good idea.*

Like taking Ambien every single night.

She smiled. I smiled back.

So, what else is up? I said. *How is your sleeping coming?*

I discontinued Zoloft, and now my therapist is concerned that the insomnia will return full force. If I wasn't comfortable with an antidepressant, he said, I should consider an anti-anxiety drug, Zanax or something, or one of the newer sleep medications.

I said nothing.

It is always delicate to balance medical/biological thinking with a more holistic or systemic approach. Ultimately it is up to the one suffering to decide what is most promising. The more suffering, the better medication looks.

They do work, you know, those meds—have you seen the ads? she said.

They can be very effective, and if they were prescribed by your doctor you should not discontinue them without his consent. Especially something as potent and long-acting as an antidepressant.

But I thought ...she said.

Continuing your meds and exploring insomnia as a symptom are not mutually exclusive. I said. *Actually you can get back in the spirit of sleeping easier when you are not battling a depression.*

But I am not depressed, she said.

Then you and your doctor might want to reconsider Zoloft. Together. I ventured.

No meds, she said, *instead focus on keeping the cat off me?* Cheryl could be quite snippy.

Yes—keeping Morris out of the bedroom is decidedly lower tech.

Meds are so much easier on everybody, she said.

No whining in front of the door all night? Even cats like them better, I agreed. *How about that for a new pitch for Pfizer?*

And no having to cut back on Merlot, or giving up late night news, or changing my whole schedule around to eat earlier. Nobody eats at seven unless you've got to get the kiddies to bed. I can't even meet my regulars for dinner on that schedule.

All sound sleepers, I ventured.

All of them sleep-challenged, she said; *drinkers by your standards and Ambien-aficionados every single one of them. You know what my friend Jen said when I mentioned that I'd been seeing a sleep doctor?*

What?

"Why? I LOVE my Ambien." Then she made bedroom-eyes and said: "Wouldn't go nighty-night without it."

So, doctor, what do YOU think? Cheryl wanted me to take sides.

Jen and millions of others, I said. *How come you are different?*

I always prided myself on being independent, and I hate the feeling that I might get hooked.

Including taking Zoloft?

Especially taking Zoloft.

35

Have you ever looked-up Zoloft in the PDR? Or went on the Internet to check on its contraindications?

And I would find what?

You would find that many antidepressants have insomnia listed as a side effect.

Really? So why prescribe it?

So far there is nothing really dependable on the market, and people who can't sleep are often anxious and depressed. So their doctors want to give them SOMETHING. On the other hand, there have been reports that some people have been doing odd things while under the influence of Ambien. The newer drugs have not been around long and widely enough to be sure there is no night eating, walking, driving ...

What about addiction? Cheryl asked.

Depends on whom you ask, I said. *There is more than one definition of addictiveness. The one drug companies use exonerates their products.*

What is the other?

Falling hopelessly in love with your drug of choice, I suggested.

I think I could get off Ambien if I decided to do it, and I don't think I have a disease.

Maybe a malaise, then, I suggested, *a culturally, socially accepted malaise with serious, oftentimes devastating side effects.*

What do you mean?

Well, there are as many fatalities due to sleep deprivation as there are due to alcohol. People eat more when they are sleep deprived, drink more, are at higher risk for obesity, diabetes, heart attacks; they bark at their loved ones and abuse the ones that work for them, they have word-retrieval issues and eventually suffer from memory losses comparable to those of pre-dementia.

Cheryl held up a hand. *I know all that. That's why I am here.*

Ready to go back to work then?

I guess. Yes.

How is the writing coming?

What is it with you and writing? It came out un-characteristically sharp.

Had a bad night?

I had bad days, and then I had bad nights.

How very astute, I said.

What?

Bad days make for bad nights, more often than not.

You want to do something about your "bad nights," as in insomnia, start doing something about your bad days.

I can't.

You are doomed.

I am not doomed; but I HAD to see my mother, it's been months! And I HAD to hang with these rich alums, and I HAD to answer my two hundred and fifty e-mails when I got back, and when I get back to work after chatting with you, I HAVE to write that report, and tomorrow night I HAVE to go to the board meeting, and make a presentation. She massaged her eyes and temples with both hands. *Jeez,* she said.

Sleep deprived, I said.

This is terrible! Cheryl stared at me.

About the writing, I ventured. *All these thoughts and insights that surfaced today, all those valuable connections you made came because you expressed yourself. You got stuff from the inside, slowed it down, contained it in words, and put it out. That's what writing can do. As a writer you get a chance to have in-sight.*

I had lots of insights in my life, Cheryl said.

The map is not the territory, I said. *Marshall McLuhan, I think. It is one thing to have an insight and quite another to live by it.*

I WANT TO SLEEP

COMMENTARY

If things go well in therapy, there will also be some predictable straining. We want to feel better; not get more depressing and tedious projects to deal with. Looking at established habits, especially our not-so-useful ones, is depressing. We all like to think of ourselves as more evolved than we really are. Taking baby steps toward recovery is dreary and often slow to reward.

For Cheryl to decide that she did not want to go the pathology route was a huge and decisive step. Getting medicated for a disease often suggests that we have no control—yet another scary thought, unless you take solace in delegating responsibility. A responsibility that might be misplaced. A recent British study suggests that long-term sleep medication users have brain-wave patterns virtually indistinguishable from those of chronic, untreated insomniacs.

Socially speaking, Cheryl's attempts to get support from friends had been unsuccessful so far, and now she wondered if she soon would be out of the loop. People have gone back to bad habits for less. I believe, though, her battle with cancer had made her an extra-determined fighter.

Cheryl is crossing over into behaviors that are no longer covered by *been there, done that* Seriously monitoring her alcohol intake? Going to bed earlier and getting up early enough for a decent breakfast? Saying no to pets, and friends who want to go partying way past bedtime? Setting limits in a work environment that rewards people like her? People who can be relied on to 'step up to the plate,' sacrifice personal preferences, and remain cheerful when used and abused by corporate priorities?

This is not what she had bargained for when she came to a 'sleep doctor'. All she really wanted was advice on getting some decent and reliable sleep so she could get on with her life as is. NOT change her life so that she could get some decent reliable sleep. People with serious, long-standing sleep problems find it hard to hear that truth: *You will have to accommodate sleep. Sleep will not accommodate you.*

Her resistance to writing seems to be almost universal. But then, our writing has forever been judged and criticized; under ordinary circumstances writing is almost by definition a way to make ourselves known to OTHERS—a scary and rejection-fraught process. Therapeutic writing is something different altogether. We are not performing on stage; we are visiting with ourselves. This kind of writing is a powerful tool to watch our typically invisible thought-habits show up on a page. One way to get our ambivalence out—and there always is ambivalence—is to write dialogues. One of the most frequently voiced objections to 'showing up on the page' is the assertion that *nothing comes to mind. I am drawing a blank.*

Our minds are never empty, let me assure you.

Write: *I can't think of anything. I can't think of a darned thing! This is stupid.*

You don't know if it is stupid unless you tried it.

I AM trying it and nothing happens.

What do you want to see happening?

I don't know; SOMETHING

Well, something is.

Like what?

You are writing, and doing good.

This is it?

Yes, this is it. Whatever you happen to think is coming out on the page.

And that is supposed to help me/

Having a listener always helps.

Session 4

Cheryl canceled her next appointment. The college she worked for had gone into its annual fund raising frenzy, and she could not take time off. In her recorded message she said she had had some interesting dreams, and that she had written them down in her sleep book. It was almost two months later when she called me for another session. She apologized and assured me that the hiatus had nothing whatsoever to do with the work we had been doing.

How kind of her. If Cheryl would afford the same consideration to her own feelings, there would be hope indeed.

How is your sleeping? I was curious; a lot of time had passed.

Funny you should ask.

It is a true joy to work with a person with a good sense of humor. And not only a joy, it is also a great predictor for therapeutic success. Humor requires a kind of mental distancing. So does looking at oneself from an unfamiliar perspective.

I have good nights, and I have had some really bad nights, Cheryl said. *But I think the nature of my bad nights has changed.*

Mmhm ...

I still wished I could sleep longer, fall asleep faster, wake up more rested—most of the time, anyway—but I am no longer afraid of going to bed.

That is fantastic.

It really is, she said. *I had avoided going to bed for many years; I don't think I told you how bad it had gotten. Now, when I can't fall asleep, I take out my trusty sleep book—* she gave me a conspiratorial smile—*and have a chat with myself. It's not so bad. Last month I forgot to pack the book when I had to go to Chicago, and I really missed it.*

It removes you from the misery of obsessive doubting and blaming.

And puts me in the presence of a much gentler person,

Cheryl smiled.

A part of yourself you had not been familiar with?

I am familiar with that part, Cheryl said, *I just never benefit from it ... her.*

Some people get confused by whom they are writing to, I said.

I am not, Cheryl smiled, *I pretend to write to YOU.*

What a creative mind you have, I said. *Is this the first time you made your mind work FOR you instead of having it haunt and harass you?*

She took a while to think about that.

I believe it is. Intentionally, anyway. My mind has served me well, especially professionally—not always personally, though.

Have your friends noticed anything different about you?

As a matter of fact, they have. They see me as having calmed down, and now they wonder when I am going to change jobs.

I raised my eyebrows in surprise.

I just can't get into that frenzy anymore with as much abandon as we all used to. We used to go crazy, and kind of thrive on the hubbub this time of the year. If that should turn out to be a job requirement, I am thinking about calling in some old chips and start doing what I really want to do.

What is that? I asked.

I always wanted to get involved in Fair Trade activities.

That is quite a change! Maybe your co-workers are a bit envious, I ventured.

I thought about that, and it brings me to something I wanted to ask you. Our health department occasionally sponsors in-house staff seminars. The last one was on how to make stress work for you instead of against you.

How do you do that? I asked.

Can't help you there, she said—*didn't go. Anyway—would you be at all interested in doing something on sleep?*

Do you think your administrators would appreciate that? They like you guys driven. I smiled.

I did conduct that workshop on a weekend in January.

The college had opened enrollment to students as well. In a planning session, Sarah, the dean of students, told me that by far the largest number of student dropouts was due do sleep deprivation. That had taken me by surprise. How did they know? It was by implication, she told me. The students themselves, in this all women's college, did not use those terms. They were just chronically tired, prone to mononucleosis and upper respiratory distress. When asked about their schedules, they said that classes started too early in the morning and Monday's shouldn't be so heavy. They objected to papers being due in the beginning of the week because nobody should be expected to work over the weekend. Parties started as early as Thursday, and often didn't get under way until eleven or twelve at night. Academic performance suffered badly. Eating disorders were the norm. Very few students ever showed up for breakfast. Only women in competitive sports seemed to fare better. Coaches insisted on early workouts and enforced no-drinking rules, especially before meets. After two semesters of burning the candle at both ends, an ever-increasing number of students felt they couldn't "handle the workload," and returned home.

Not surprisingly, a fair number of parents questioned the school's commitment to student welfare. They had just spent tens of thousands of dollars, and now their girls were dropping out with nothing much to show for it. The school, on the other hand, made a case for "helping people grow up" rather than infantilizing them. Parents felt their money should buy more guidance.

If sleep deprivation was an identifiable factor, I ventured, couldn't the school step in and do something about it? Like, for example, enforce sleep-conducive schedules?—if not on the whole campus, than maybe in selected dormitories? Lights out by eleven? No loud parties or pizza deliveries, and an agreed-upon closed-door policy? Drop outs were a bad thing all around, right? If the school didn't intervene, who should?

People looked at me as if I had time-warped from an earlier century.

Everybody would be better off, I argued. The women would get a chance to sleep, the campus would be safer, academics would improve, professors and parents alike would welcome a return to the stated purpose of higher education, the townspeople—increasingly intolerant of rowdy late-night behavior—might look upon the college-kids more kindly. All it would take was an informed, firm proposal to the student council.

Sounded like win-win to me.

Impossible.

We are not dealing here with little kids, a somewhat defensive administrator pointed out. Students might even riot, as they had in a neighboring town when some of the frat houses were closed down. *Too much interference in people's personal freedom. Counter to the college's mission of turning out responsible adults.* My tenure was not at stake, so I just acted incredulous: *Are you for real? You have a bad situation; you know what the problem is; you have the means to initiate changes but you are not pursuing the obvious next steps?*

What had just been put into academic policy was the same attitude that—much less obviously so—my sleep-challenged patients exhibited: *I don't want to hear about uncomfortable and unpopular changes. What we pay you for is expert advice at making undesirable symptoms go away.*

I don't want to stop drinking, what can you do for my hangovers?

I WANT TO SLEEP

I don't want to put the brakes on my runaway life—any suggestions on how to rest up for it more efficiently?

Only the nurse practitioner who headed the small in-house clinic looked at me thoughtfully.

When and if these kids graduate, they will fit seamlessly into any corporate culture, which expects interns to work late nights and weekends, have lunch at their desk, override exhaustion with double lattes, and force mental oblivion with alcohol.

One by one, almost to the person, people came up to me afterwards and expressed their concern for a development that they felt unprepared to confront. The medical staff implied that they actually supported student dropouts despite the college's tuition-driven policies. Their reason? The risks of serious medical implications and personal safety concerns were just too high with chronically sleep-deprived kids; and they were afraid of litigation.

As it turned out, the administrators had underestimated their students' commitment to a more reasonable life-management. The kids expressed significant interest in a sleep-friendly dormitory but much less curiosity in the sleep-enhancing techniques that I had come prepared to teach.

There is anecdotal wisdom in many therapeutic paradigms that patients have something to teach their therapists. If that came to be a dominant feature, fee arrangements would have to be renegotiated. Nevertheless, it is always wise to be open and have one's pre-conceived notions enhanced. As in this instance: Until I spoke to those young women, it had not occurred to me how much of a social, collective dimension there can be to sleeping. *I* was advocating something along the lines of a dark and quiet environment. *They* wanted to be sure everyone concerned was collectively "into sleeping." If it was understood that people would settle down for sleep at a certain time, if everyone in the dorm were on the same page, they thought they'd have no problem sleeping whatsoever. *"Oh-my-God,"* would they welcome it.

Conversely—not that anybody had quite put it that way—the students made themselves stay up with all its torturous consequences, because everyone else did. To be socially marginalized was worse than jeopardizing a semester's work of studies—and incidentally one's health.

I wondered how much of this dynamic was gender-specific. I also wondered how much this need to belong affected the sleep patterns of some of the people who came to see me.

COMMENTARY

Cheryl was someone who could no longer bridge the gap between waking and going towards sleep. She also belonged to a group who had accepted sleep deprivation as part of their identity. Her presleep efforts were one performance failure after the other. For a high performer to fail so miserably night after night, at a task that is as elementary as it is crucial, had become cause for self-doubt, and eventually self-loathing. I know for a fact that many people, especially successful people, many of them women, suffer the same fate.

I say women because men as a rule sleep easier. I believe this has to do with a different attitude about caring and sensitivity.

I can't be bothered; or: *What has that got to do with me? Let them worry about it! I don't care. Hey, that's not MY problem.*

Those are almost classic male lines. If you can clear your presleep time of bother and whatever problems there are— they are not yours, then there will indeed be much less tossing and turning. *All my husband needs,* complained one woman to me, *is a couch.*

What worked for Cheryl was a subtle shift in focus. It wasn't anymore about getting enough sleep so she could stay on an unmodified course. She began to hear her nightly distress as a plea: *Please ease up on me! I am being sold out here.*

She could not—nobody can—sleep on demand; but she could accomplish some sleep-enabling tasks. That they were hard to do—keeping a sleep journal, modifying her daily routines, saying no to some obvious sleep-deterrents—might have actually helped engage her serious and diligent mind. THOSE were things she could tackle, inconvenient as they might be. As her confidence returned, bedtime was no longer the predictable ordeal it had been for years. Bedtime had become an opportunity to think about Cheryl. Her helplessness and hopelessness gradually yielded to intentional remedial steps, and since Cheryl was a realist, she did not despair when results were not instantaneous or always predictable. She also developed a subtle appreciation for those unscheduled nightly gifts of private time. Some of her most cherished inspirations had surfaced there.

The young women I met in that college workshop were at an earlier stage of insomnia. They had not yet—most of them anyway—unlearned crossing over into unconsciousness and could not strictly speaking be called insomniacs, despite severe symptoms of sleep deprivation. They still could drop off to sleep unaided despite noise levels and physical inconvenience—but not without collective consent. Even sleeping in crowded airports or next to wailing babies still worked for them. It's what college kids do. At school, though, they prevented themselves from sleeping for mainly social reasons. My concern is that eventually their sleep abilities will atrophy from disuse, a fate many of our other mental and physical abilities share. If you don't use it you lose it. Going to sleep is a skill, as those who have lost it can appreciate. After years of forcing wakefulness and neglecting going to sleep when their bodies are desperate to do so, these students risk ending up like Cheryl.

MICHAEL was referred by his internist.

There is nothing wrong with me physically, Dr. Ross says. He wants me to talk to you and get your opinion on maybe going to a sleep clinic.

This is how Michael introduced himself.

He was in his early thirties, an accountant turned schoolteacher. He was married, and they expected a baby later that fall.

Michael took good care of himself; he worked out daily, didn't drink, didn't smoke—*never have*—he said. He and his wife, an art teacher, were vegetarians; there was family money that took the worry out of family planning. About three months ago Michael developed an inability to go to sleep. All he could think of was jet lag. The symptoms appeared after returning from a trip to Europe and never had subsided since.

What have you done about it so far? I asked.

First I took some melatonin as they say you should with jet lag, Michael said. *Then, when that didn't work, Dr. Ross gave me a prescription for Lunesta.*

And that doesn't help you sleep either?

It does knock me out, but I don't like taking it all the time. There's got to be something wrong, you know? All of a sudden I can't sleep? That doesn't make any sense. I've never had a problem before.

Jet lag can do that. I said, *but melatonin is only reliable when taken in the right dosage.*

I took 3 mgs four hours before going to bed. It seemed to help first ... he trailed off, discouraged.

Some recent British studies suggest, I said, *that melatonin is more effective for a longer period of time when taken in much lower doses; a tenth of what you took, maybe.*

It only comes in 3 mg capsules, he said.

I know, I nodded.

And the sleep clinic? I asked.

It seems like a logical next step, Michael said. *Maybe there is something wrong, you know, with my brain; they probably could tell.*

Sleep clinics are most effective in diagnosing and treating sleep apnea. I said.

I don't have that; I don't even snore, he said. *Jess would have told me, I am sure. Where do you think I should go from here?*

You are talking about going to a sleep clinic? I asked.

Yes, Michael said *the whole ball of wax.*

Call them and ask to talk to an insomnia-specialist. Insist they tell you what they can do for people who do not have apnea.

Okay. I'll do that. But what do YOU think?

I think you are getting more anxious as time goes on. Tell me what's on your mind when you can't sleep?

Well, the baby, of course, and if I am going to be a good father. I think I will...Then they gave me an all-new course to teach at school. Some kind of introduction into business. I don't even know where to start.

Help me with the math, I said. *The baby is due when?*

Well, she was conceived in Europe, he said; *our due date is end of August, beginning of September.* Then, in anticipation of my next comment: *I am not worried about THAT. I am excited! We are both really looking forward to having a family.*

Excitement is a form of agitation, I said.

I gave Michael some homework. I wanted to know what happened in the four hours or so before he went to bed, and if there had been any changes in their routine since the Europe trip. Other than the trip itself, of course.

Michael brought a legal pad to the next session, detailing day by day, or night by night rather, what their evenings looked like.

What struck me was the number of movies they watched. As subscribers to Netflix, they watched one or two movies every night; tuned in to the 11o'clock news, checked their e-mail one last time, then went to bed with something to read.

Since they had come back from Europe, Jess, Michael's wife, tended to fall asleep during the last movie (as she had on the plane), then drowsily went upstairs, started reading and barely made it through the first five pages.

While you?

While I am still wide awake, too worked up to read and too exhausted to sleep. Michael said.

Too worked up? I asked.

Well, yes. I am a not much of a tough guy, Michael seemed apologetic. *Movies can be kind of heavy, especially when you watch really good ones. We belong to a discussion group, and when we get together with friends all we talk about are movies.*

It's almost like being back in New York, I said.

Exactly, Michael said, pleased that I understood.

This was going to be difficult.

Like many people Michael did not know that—as far as sleep is concerned—agitation is agitation. There is no "good upset" or "bad upset."

These days, 'good books' and 'good movies' are almost by definition upsetting and emotionally wrenching. We live in a culture that thrives on extravagant excitement, buildup, and graphic emotional distress. People say it makes them "feel alive." What it makes them feel is wired. We are in danger of confusing being wired with feeling alive.

Fortunately for us there is reliable bio feedback: the more confusion the more insomnia.

Many of my patients are hooked on being worked up, and media exploit and push the adrenalin addiction. Sleep, on the other hand, does not thrive on distress or even excitement. Upsetting movies, books, conversations, e-mails, or marital discussions trigger ancient biological warnings. Sleep is primal, and a vulnerable state; alerting your system even for the most laudable of causes will cost you sleep.

I WANT TO SLEEP

You are hooked on agitants, I said to Michael

Agitants? he asked.

Yes, agitating stimuli. Adrenalin; mental coffee. Cortisol.

I don't drink coffee, Michel said

You guzzle excitement, mentally agitating input. By the time you close your eyes your brain is on speed.

My brain is always on speed, Michael said.

Well, it went on overdrive when you were overtired, overstimulated, overextended on your way back from France.

I need to calm down, Michael said. *I know that.*

That's not a sleep problem; I said *that's a waking problem.*

A waking problem? What's a waking problem?

It's called S.O.L.D. I call it SOLD; I should say; it's not an official disease.

What does it stand for?

Stimulus Overload Disorder.

You got a cure for it too?

Of course, I said. *It's called 'cold turkey'.*

You are not kidding, Michael said, taken aback.

Michael, as it turned out, had taken to the word 'agitant'—also, of course, not a real word. But it evoked something in him that helped classify mental exposure. He had been an accountant after all. He started scanning his evenings for *agitants* and, not surprisingly, found many. In his following sessions Michael wanted to talk about school stress. I was the one who had to bring up sleeping.

It's certainly better, he said. *But then we are going to bed much earlier. That makes me less anxious about lying awake. You know? There is less pressure to get that rest.*

'Pressure to get that rest?' Talking about an oxymoron. Is there anything you do without pressure? I asked.

I still remember Michael's slow smile: *I cook*, he said.

I have a suggestion, I offered at a later session.

We had previously met as a threesome; and Jess, I knew, was more than willing to modify their evening routines.

Since you have a baby on the way, you might want to revisit children's literature. You're going to read a lot of kids' books during the next six years.

Start with the ones you liked as a kid and read them to each other.

Like Charlotte's Web? He said.

Or: The Cricket in Time Square.

I WANT TO SLEEP

Jess really likes Winnie the Pooh.

There you go, I said.

COMMENTARY

Michael's sleeping got gradually better and improved noticeably after the couple started reading together. There is something extra unsettling about lying awake next to someone who sleeps with no trouble at all. Michael said that he and Jess now *pretty much go to sleep at the same time—give or take.* Sometimes I wonder if a couple can only afford one insomniac at a time because I have rarely heard of two people lying awake simultaneously—unless of course they were waiting for their kids to come home.

Most of the time Michael was fine now, and he had started to cook more. Preparing food superimposes slower rhythms. Marketing takes time and diligence. Having friends appreciate your bread and your pasta is rewarding. All good sleep things to do. And vegetarian meals are easier to digest.

Michael's schedule allowed mainly for weekend cooking, which proved to have an unexpected fringe benefit. Sunday nights had been the worst for sleep, as is true for many people. After all there is Monday to worry about. Especially after he had prepared a meal for friends on a Sunday night, sleeping had become a 'non-issue,' as Michael called it.

Sometime during this period, Michael made an

appointment with a newly established sleep center in town. *Just to play it safe.* The study showed no abnormal patterns.

I actually slept pretty well despite being hooked up and all, Michael reported.

I think all that professional attention comforted him.

As the pregnancy progressed, he started worrying about being kept up by the baby. Friends told horror stories, and he wanted to know if that meant his insomnia would return.

Being kept up by your baby is not insomnia, I assured him. *Something in you will know the difference between you giving yourself a hard time or the baby needing attention. Something in you will even know if it is your night to get up and change diapers or Jess's. On your night you'll wake at the first whimper—on Jess's nights you'll sleep through a full-blown wail.*

Why is that? Michael was intrigued.

I don't know, Mike, I said. *Something, somebody in us is smarter than we think.*

A recent study by the Sleep Research Center in the Department of Psychiatry at Pennsylvania State University concluded that the cause of insomnia was stress. In paraphrasing their words: You can't sleep when your hypothalamic-pituitary-adrenal axis is over activated. The resulting hyper arousal due to elevated levels of Cortisol and ACTH is dangerous if chronic. Sleep therapy therefore should aim at decreasing the level of physiological and emotional arousal and not just improve nighttime sleep.

There you have it. Just fighting your insomnia when part of the problem is stimulation pollution will not do you justice.

CHAPTER 2
I CAN'T STAY ASLEEP

LYDIA

I nterrupted sleep entails a loss of continuity. It is probably the second most frequent complaint as far as sleep problems are concerned, but fewer people seem to seek help for it than for sleep-onset insomnia.

Not everybody is afraid of going to bed. Many people fall asleep all right—with or without the help of a little something. Then, depending on the case, they wake up two or four hours later and stay awake until they might as well get up. By that time it is often too late to resort to a trusted sleep-aid. The risk of not waking up in time for work is too high. In elderly populations where this is no longer an issue people tend to be less careful, and risk stumbling and falling as a result. Hangover symptoms from drugs that have not worked themselves out of the system can seriously jeopardize physical coordination and full alertness in the morning.

People will say, *But I only took a half!* without realizing that many sedative effects are cumulative. Only half of the drug is fully metabolized when its promised effectiveness wears out. The other half gets added on to next night's pill.

These half-life effects are often the cause of serious misjudgments and misunderstandings.

Because there seems to be such a well-established tie-in between menopause and interrupted sleep, few women consider psychological help. Establishing a connection, however, and positing a causative link are not the same. There are people, situations, and cultures where insomnia is not considered a given when a woman enters menopause.

Lydia was someone who wondered about that. Now in her sixties, she had not encountered any "bad nights" until menopause. Then she woke up in sweats, uncomfortable and "bothered," as she put it. Gradually, this had become an established pattern, interrupted briefly when she went on estrogen-replacement therapy. When she decided her family history would put her at risk for breast cancer, and discontinued her medication, sleep-interruptions resumed with a vengeance.

Lydia had signed up for a sleep workshop in San Miguel de Allende, Mexico. SMA, as the cognoscenti call it, has a large enough expatriate population to ensure the viability of a small counseling/personal growth center.

When I had planned the seminar with Joseph, one of the principals, I expressed my suspicion that there might not be enough interest among all those relaxed gringos.

How much stress can one accumulate sitting around the Jardin all day, going to gallery openings at night, and then, after a few drinks at Harry's, listening to the mariachis out-fiddling each other? I had asked.

Joseph assured me that there would be plenty of sleep-challenged people, and he was right. That workshop was booked up three days after it had been advertised in the *Atencion*. It was also one of the most lively and challenging venues in my career, because the majority of participants were professionals, or ex-professionals in health-related fields.

Lydia called me a few days after the workshop and asked to see me.

I found your workshop very interesting, she said with the faintest of Texan twangs. *I am one of the people who wake up at four, almost on the dot, every night, and that's the end of that.*

Since I am down here, I said, *I too wake up at four, but for me it's the roosters and the dogs on our neighbors' roofs.*

The roosters and the dogs, she smiled. *I love them. I believe I am used to them and probably would miss them if they locked them up. There are some people who are complaining, you know.*

Not Mexicans, I said. *No, not Mexicans, of course.*

About your sleep pattern: A lot of perimenopausal women have very similar complaints. I followed-up. *This form of insomnia is thought to be caused by estrogen withdrawal. In women, anyway.*

I know. I got relief as soon as I went on replacement therapy. Then it all came back when I decided against continuing. Lydia said.

Was there anything in my presentation that made you think I could be of help?

She smiled apologetically. *Actually*, she said, *it was something Lupe my housekeeper said.*

I was intrigued.

Lupe has been with me for over fifteen years, and by now there is very little we don't know about each other.

I nodded.

Well, Lupe says that she does not know anybody in her village or in her family who has insomnia. She was polite about it, but I could tell she had her "crazy gringo" face on: "People pay money to learn how to sleep?" She asked how much I paid.

Lydia laughed.

Insomnia sometimes seems to be in the eye of the beholder, I said. *I remember a New Yorker cartoon where a bleary eyed wife questions her husband who is watching late-night TV. "It's only insomnia," he says, "if it is no fun".*

Lydia agreed. *I actually wondered about that myself,* she said. *Lupe's family lives outside Dolores. The roosters and dogs alone, not to mention donkeys and burros, will wake you up at daybreak.*

But then, I said, *there is always siesta. And it might be time to get cooking anyway.*

I WANT TO SLEEP

Out there they still do have a siesta, Lydia agreed. *Maybe they just don't call it insomnia. Lupe still takes it but she wants me to believe she needs time to read her Bible. "Una siestita" she calls it.*

I then asked Lydia about her own siesta, and she laughed and said she didn't have any.

Why not? You are living in Mexico, and you don't have a siesta? That's one of the reasons to go to Mexico in the first place!

I am taking afternoon classes at the Bellas Artes—*same people, same teacher now for years and years,* Lydia said. *We meet at two.*

All gringos, I bet.

Lydia smiled.

Waking up too early in the morning is not that much of a big deal when you can make up with a snooze in the afternoon, I said.

Aren't you supposed to sleep only at night? She asked. *I seem to remember reading somewhere that we all should aim for a good night's sleep, and even if we can't do that, we shouldn't take naps. Because if you take naps, you'll be liable to not sleeping at night.*

I know, I said. *It's in all the professional sleep-advice columns all over the Internet. My hunch is these guys never traveled outside the US. The only people who lose out from taking naps are employers. And sometimes I am not even sure about that.*

But there is research, Lydia said. *It's the only reason why I take some medication. Not all the time, of course. But people do need to sleep.*

What do you take? I asked.

I break off a corner of some Ambien when I need to be on the ball, as they say; not a very nice expression, I am afraid.

At four in the morning? I asked. *Lydia, this is how people break their hips.*

I don't take enough to have me go stumbling about, if that is what you mean. And I wouldn't do it at all if medical research ... She trailed off.

If there was research that proved that afternoon naps are essential for a person's mental and physical health—would you do it?

I might, I'd certainly feel more right about it, Lydia said.

I'll make a bet with you that within a year or so someone will scientifically prove that naps are not bad, and can have some bona fide health benefits.

I am not sure I should wait another year. Lydia was half serious. *I did fall once when I had to get up, you know. Nothing serious, though.*

Tell you what, I said, *you start taking siestas, two hours minimum, and tell your friends you're following doctor's orders.*

I am sick of trying to paint the Parochia (SMA's most photogenic church) anyway, Lydia said.

We had one more meeting that spring because I had to go back to cold New England. It was a chance meeting in San Miguel's central park—the Jardin—not so chancy, really when everyone is there at least once a day anyway.

Lydia was in the company of a short, prim woman in a starched white blouse who was trying to manage an incongruously undisciplined little fluffy dog.

Dr. Haug, Lydia said, but did not introduce me to the woman, I took to be Lupe.

The two o'clock painting class disbanded. We are now meeting for bridge at five. I also decided that it was too hot to play tennis in the afternoon. Don't you agree?

I would still be napping, but I am sure you are right, I said.

She indulged me in my nap joke.

I am still waking up at four, though, Lydia said. *Did I tell you I am a birder?*

I don't believe you did.

Most of my friends are birders; we are planning to go up to the botanical garden one of these mornings.

67

Excellent, I said. *Not much birding to be done at siesta time anyway, I suppose.*

The birds, Lupe said, *they have siesta too.*

I like Lydia's story because it reminds us that healing is not the same as making something undesirable go away. That is an important perspective when dealing with a multitude of sleep-adverse situations. Making lemonade when you are dealt lemons is much more than just making do. It is an amazing creative turn around. A former liability is transformed into an asset. If you happen to be a birder, early morning up in the Botanical Garden is as good as it gets.

Lydia's inability to go back to sleep at four in the morning did not get better.

When I met her a year later, though, she was no longer sleep deprived. Siesta had become a sacred institution in her old colonial home. Shutters were closed from one to three and she put on her pajamas.

Something else had happened as well, and I believe it had to do with the scaling back of her sleep-deprived chronic fatigue. Lydia had been a pediatric nurse in a former life. After her husband, a cardiologist, died, she moved to San Miguel permanently but never went back to her profession. About three months after our last meeting, she was invited to a christening in Lupe's village. The need for basic pediatric care had not been lost on her. Without the legal concerns of our own litigious society, she soon became a regular consultant to local midwives and the overworked staff of a remote rural clinic. Soon her well-to-do friends were raising funds for an on-site nurse who would serve three neighboring villages.

COMMENTARY

It seems to me that many people with Lydia's affliction are trying to resign themselves to their fate—and for good reason. There are few remedies that I have heard people agree on. Oftentimes it is too late to try medication, or too early, rather, in the morning, to attempt a safe drug-induced sleep. Most women I have talked to help themselves with teas and herbs. Some of them are home-grown. An elderly nurse told me that she extracted wild lettuce juice, which works as a mild sedative. How about just eating it for dinner? Others have hop tinctures by their bedside, or valerian pills (Valerian takes several weeks to become effective). A significant number of women swear by preparations given to them by Chinese herbalists.

At least I had a couple of hours, the not-so-lucky ones tell themselves. While sleep-onset difficulties rarely get better by themselves (anxiety metastasizes), not being able go to back to sleep sometimes works itself out. More often than not people manage to make life style adjustments, like going to bed earlier, changing eating habits, napping, or talking on the phone. Several of my patients get up, write a couple of pages, and report having an easier time re-entering sleep. Some have down-loaded books, put their ipods on a timer, and fall asleep listening to stories. I wish I had more data on men, but men don't go to therapy as a rule. I wonder, for example if male menopause, *andropause,* has a similar effect on late-midlife men's sleeping patterns. If so, would a diet high in phytoestrogens—as in soy products—alleviate the symptoms?

We have documents dating back hundreds of years that mention a "first" and a "second" sleep. People would wake up in the middle of the night, socialize some, and then go back to sleep for another installment. The many forms of siesta-like accommodations suggest that humans might never have been designed to get eight solid hours in one stretch and then be forced to stay awake continuously for another sixteen. The truth is nobody, even good sleepers, sleeps continuously. Sleep studies show that humans wake up—briefly—many more times than we remember. Good sleepers have no problem going right back to sleep. They actually relish the reentry. Troubled sleepers stay awake. It turns out that good sleeping is not the same as sleeping continuously. It means being able to come and go with ease.

Walt Whitman (1819-1892) seems to have been a good sleeper—not because he didn't have wakeful periods but because he relished them:

> *This is thy hour O Soul, thy free flight into the wordless,*
> *Away from books, away from art, the day erased, the lessons done.*
> *Thee fully forth emerging, silent, grazing, pondering the themes thou lovest best, night, sleep, death and the stars.*

"A Clear Midnight"

Instead of going Oh no! I like to believe Whitman sat down and wrote this poem when he woke up in the middle of the night.

My hunch is that situational factors also play a role when people wake up too early and can't go back to sleep. One of them is obvious: daylight is dawning, and they won't get any help from the body's melatonin output, which is triggered by dusk. With jet lag, our circadian rhythms have been disrupted, and we wake up at the wrong time. If that happens with some frequency, the body loses its sense of timing and sleep comes too early or too late.

I wondered how professional pilots on international cargo runs handle their sleeping needs. The answer was simple and unanimous: *sleep anytime and anywhere you get an opportunity.* Medication is out, so grab that shut-eye any chance you get.

But there are also other disruptions, oftentimes of a traumatic nature, that threaten and jeopardize sleep continuity on deeper levels. Menopause is such a breach of continuity; a divorce, a re-location, empty-nest syndrome, early retirement, a life-threatening disease. It is especially evident in older people, whose lives are disrupted on all levels. A long-term spouse might have died, living in a partial care facility might have become necessary; body parts may have given out, careers have come to an end. It is devastating to wake up and find the other side of the bed empty. During sleep we forgot the loss. Now it hits home again and even years later we can be as unprepared for the shock as if the person had gone only yesterday. Waking oneself up early is one way of coping because it is less traumatic. This way morning cannot catch us by surprise. I believe this is why some people report this kind of waking up as having almost no burdensome transitions.

One moment I am asleep, the next I am awake. Eyes open,

just like that, Lydia once said.

I also believe there is a substantially underreported medicinal use of alcohol for sleep induction; especially with older people who don't have to show up for work bright and early, live alone, and can leave the rest of the world none the wiser.

Cheryl owned up to two glasses of wine a night. Another woman, a successful real-estate professional, who contacted me for phone-consultations consumed one bottle a night to "help her sleep" and more when she had had a "bad day." Alcohol truncates sleep and also might play a role in those early awakenings. Then there is the hard-to-track use of antihistamines and cold medications. Patients often report that they stumbled on their sleep-enabling side effects by sheer accident. Others caught on after a pediatrician prescribed them for their kids' sleep problems.

Where men's wakefulness is concerned, there is always BPH, benign prostatic hyperplasia, and the urge to urinate. Allan used palmetto extract and swore by it, even though a recent study had declared it ineffective. *Who paid for the study?* he wanted to know. I had no idea.

ALLAN

Allan, one of the small number of male clients in my practice, wanted help with going back to sleep. He is a successful 65-year-old businessman, a former competitive sailor who is proud of his fitness.

He had heard of hypnosis as an effective way to induce

sleep, and being a firm believer in affirmations, wanted to know if I could help him. There really was nothing else bothering him in his life, he said, other than that deplorable trend of waking up earlier and earlier in the morning.

As part of my intake procedure, I checked on potential medical concerns. His annual health check had been uneventful as usual, even though his blood pressure seemed to be creeping up and needed monitoring. His PSAs (prostate specific antigens) were slightly up but then, his doctor had said, a larger prostate makes more antigens. Allan ate well, rarely consumed alcohol, never smoked, and exercised regularly. I commented on his habit of clearing his throat, and he told me that he was a bit nervous.

How long had this getting up early been going on? I asked.

Forever, Allan laughed. *In my younger years it served me well. I was in the office before anyone else; the early bird, you know?*

When did it become troublesome? I wanted to know.

Really troublesome? After I moved back home.

Well, he continued after a pause that I did not fill, *I doubt it has anything to do with my sleeping but I might as well tell you.*

The story that followed was long, moving, and painful.

Allan had separated from his wife early in their marriage, and brought up their two children by himself. His wife gradually confronted her alcoholism, but they had lived separate lives for most of the past thirty years. Both had been with several partners on and off. After the kids had grown up, Allan and his wife decided to buy a house in the country and try living together. While he was still traveling on business, things went well. He loved his wife and admired her style and worldly flair. As he spent more time at home, he noticed that she had resumed having a glass or two of wine for dinner. Being a successful graduate of many an Alanon meeting, he didn't say anything. But it bothered him very much. When she had been drinking she became belligerent, wanted to know if he was still in contact with former partners, and accused him of alienating the kids from her. She also snored *significantly*, as Allan put it, but vehemently refused to let him sleep in another bedroom.

"We might as well not be married," she says when I tell her that I need to get an undisturbed good night's rest. I don't think she would leave me just for sleeping somewhere else, but I can't even think of living in that big house by myself.

It is hard to get a good night's rest when someone snores next to you. I said.

Somehow her snoring is not so bad in the early morning hours, but by then, of course, I am awake.

People who sleep with a snorer sometimes stay awake anticipating the next snoring episode, I said. *Somehow it seems more tolerable to be prepared than to be jolted awake again.*

That's true, Allan said; then, with a wry smile: *plus I can check up on her.*

I wasn't sure what he meant and told him so.

No, no, I am not worried about her getting sick or something. It's more like making sure she is still there.

You are afraid she might take off?

Allan shrugged his shoulders. *She has, at times.*

As always, towards the end of any initial session, I sing the praises of writing.

Keep minutes, I said. *A lot can get lost in the flow of a session. Go over what we covered today. Highlight things that seem relevant to your sleep problems.*

We didn't get to do much hypnotizing, I said, as he prepared to leave.

That's quite all right, Allan said, *I enjoyed our little talk.*

One physical sleep component with vast symbolic implications has to do with getting enough air.

Getting relief for physical discomfort is what every person with chronic or intractable pain prays for. Not being able to breathe is just as formidable an enemy to sleep. There are several things that can produce instant anxiety. One of them is not getting enough air. Breathing is vital, and we refer to it in sayings like: "I couldn't breathe in this relationship", or "coming up for air." Something can "take our breath away" or "knock the air out of us." Since sleep is so very anxiety-sensitive, even the physical difficulty of drawing breath through an obstructed nose can wake you up. So can postnasal drip if it reduces air flow.

Allan kept clearing his throat a lot; by now initial anxiety could no longer be held responsible; so I brought it up again.

It's just postnasal drip, he said.

How long have you had it? I pursued.

It seems to have gotten worse in the past year or so, Allan said. *First it was just a matter of getting a cold; now I seem to have it all the time.*

Does it force you to switch from breathing through your nose to breathing with your mouth?

At night? Allan asked.

Mmhm.

I can't breathe through my mouth. It makes me snore.

How do you know that? I asked.

Believe me, my wife lets me know.

She wakes you up?

You bet.

I WANT TO SLEEP

So you try breathing through your nose even though it is obstructed? I asked.

It's not so bad, Allan said.

Did you by any chance change your diet in the past couple of years? I asked.

I became a vegetarian. Why do you ask?

I used to work in New York, I said, *and a lot of my early clients were young performing artists. From them I learned that you should never eat dairy a couple of days before you go on stage.*

Why not?

It seems to produce enough mucus to jeopardize your voice. Mucus, postnasal drip, stuffed nose, lying on your back—a recipe for tough sleeping.

Are you saying I'd sleep better if I went off dairy products?

It would be worth checking out, don't you think? Suppose you did develop a sensitivity to dairy, and part of your stuffy nose and your postnasal drip—especially if it is clear—is because you eat a lot of cheese.

It is amazing how sleeping, bad sleeping, and our subsequent quest for improvement frequently come back to seemingly unrelated lifestyle changes. Allan had become a vegetarian to please his wife. In all likelihood his postnasal drip was aggravated by this change in diet.

No—this is certainly not the main reason for Allan's insomnia nor is it the only one: Switching to goat cheese, though, could bring some relief. After all, the journey of one thousand miles starts with one seemingly inconsequential step in the right direction. That still will leave him with a snoring wife who feels strongly that couples should sleep together—and if not actually sleep, then at least go through the motions of sharing the marital bed. Easy for her to say. Snorers might not sleep as well as they could, but they do sleep.

Allan kept seeing me for a long time. He said he loved his wife but clearly was unhappy with the living arrangements. He talked about feeling trapped. Every now and then I brought up his initial complaint.

You haven't talked about sleeping now for several weeks. Do you get enough rest?

I am still waking up too early on occasion, he said, *then my mind gets going.*

Problems at three or four in the morning can take on insurmountable proportions, I said. *How are you managing?*

I tell myself: I've got to remember to bring this up with Siegfried.

And that helps you get back to sleep? I asked.

Not necessarily, Allan said, *but it kind of takes the wind out of its sail.*

I WANT TO SLEEP

What about the snoring?

I bought earplugs, the wax ones that swimmers use.

That works? I asked.

It works for me. We are also not sleeping in the same room most nights.

How did that happen? I asked.

Well, I finally said something about the drinking and how unpleasant things were even after one single glass. My wife took exception to that and left the dinner table.

And she does not want you sleeping with her?

All I have to do is bring up the drinking and she walks off. He smiled wryly.

Allan's focus had shifted from managing his nights to making the most of his days. He was planning on retiring early and spent extended periods of time exploring places in the south.

I wondered what had happened to his fears of being alone.

When my wife is drinking, I am alone anyway, he said.

Allan's situation is not at all atypical. What is somewhat unusual is the gender switch. It is by far more common that men object to their bedmates moving out. The symbolism seems to bode so very badly.

I remember a snoring husband joining a session for this reason alone: he was irate and hurt that I had suggested someone move to another bedroom. In this particular case there was no shortage of bedrooms, and nobody would be relegated to a lumpy couch. He was all worked up, *not being a believer in this kind of thing*—meaning psychotherapy—and wanted to let me know in no uncertain terms that I had crossed a sacred line. The symbolism of sleeping together is indeed old and powerful. Many a bedmate has sacrificed decades of good sleep to its archetypal power. As a therapist I believe in the power of symbols, and I sympathized with this gentleman's distress. The problem was, if his wife was to be believed, that he was a relentless snorer of considerable proportions. This particular episode dates back to a time when sleep clinics were few and far between and sleep apnea was something only doctors knew how to spell. Today we'd have him fitted with a mask in no time. Back then, I had to appeal to his professed love for his wife, and we agreed to tape a random night in the couple's bedroom. He could not rightly refuse this kind of evidence gathering, even though he felt pretty sure his wife was overly sensitive and had been exaggerating.

The results were truly remarkable, and to his credit, he even allowed segments to be played for fun when the kids came home for Thanksgiving. He was a big man, and he could make windows rattle. Friends sheepishly admitted that they had abstained from inviting the couple to their lakeside cottage because *nobody* was able to sleep the nights he stayed over. It has always puzzled me how snorers themselves manage to disconnect their auditory nerves. The noise right inside their own skulls must be deafening. Interestingly enough, this gentleman could even sleep through a playback of his own snoring; an experience I had hoped would allow for a change of mind as far as their sleep arrangements were concerned. What DID change his mind was his family's sympathy. He was being lauded as quite the enlightened husband when he suggested they adopt some other arrangement.

His wife's problems with sleeping did not end there, however. For months afterwards she found herself awake in the middle of the night, an occasion she utilized to read extensively and without guilt. I am not sure she got around to telling him that. Being brought up on a farm *idle hands* were frowned upon and reading was for the leisure class. Now she could read all she wanted without disturbing anybody. She considered it a luxury. We don't seem to need all our problems to go away as far as better sleeping is concerned. What we do need is a break in an otherwise hopelessly entrenched pattern. What we need is the hope that things can change.

This is a promising prospect. Maybe there never was a time when humans slept continuous, uninterrupted, wonderful sleeps—night after night. After all, there always were babies, coughs, roosters, and dogs—enough disruptions anyway to make a good night's sleep something special. Maybe there also were not so many snorers, because snoring seems to be associated with another recent cultural phenomenon: increasing obesity.

Why then our epidemic insomnia concerns, especially among the upwardly mobile?

One reason might be that many people can no longer *afford* to have good days and bad days, good nights and bad nights. Like machines, they have to deliver top performance day after day. If sleeping is seen as a performance, however, insomnia will increasingly affect other vulnerable members of society: adolescents and even babies. Treating sleep as yet another personal achievement, or a consumer commodity does not work. Another reason for wide-spread sleep problems is, I believe, the result of unremitting, sixteen to eighteen hours worth of audiovisual overstimulation.

I have found that better sleep rarely requires radical changes. What it does require is a sense of hope for improvement, the relief that comes from breaking the power of a previously invincible pattern. Unfortunately, culturally condoned anti-sleep patterns have become so pervasive that there is little hope in sight. *Sleep,* one young woman told me *is for losers.* It is hard to sleep when you feel hopeless and trapped.

COMMENTARY

It is rare in my experience to meet a person whose sleep problems are not wake-problems. Bad days seem to make for bad nights. That is an unwelcome message for most insomniacs, who would like it to be the other way around. "Bad days" do not necessarily mean rough days, or difficult days, but destabilizing, emotionally upsetting, agitated, over stimulated days—days that seem to ensnare our minds in their clutches and follow us home. While we are awake we have learned to deal with obsessing by moving on and changing the subject; at night this option peters out and we are alone with our rattled, unprotected selves. Some people, oftentimes men, have learned to shrug off whatever might dent their protective armor. Thousands of years of breeding soldiers might have given rise to extra thick skins. While this is difficult for relationships, it does wonders for sleeping. Sensitivity might be desirable in a mate, but it translates into "thin skin" on a personal level. Its permeable boundaries jeopardize sleep. Sensitive responsiveness makes for an unprotected, unsafe, and anxious inner world.

For sleep to take over, we need to *feel* safe. Having a thicker skin makes for safer boundaries. I have met men in couples therapy who felt completely safe in their relationships as they were only months away from a divorce.

Vice versa, I have met women who felt that good sleeping was a sign of inexcusable insensitivity, given the state our world is in.

Allan was a sensitive man. It was how he gained the trust of his clients, and his responsiveness to their needs had made him a fortune. He also had been scared of being alone all his life. People took to him because he knew how to meet their requirements. He met their needs so they would not leave him.

Talking to me was a big relief for Allan, and there is hardly a better sleep tonic than feeling relieved. He wanted to be hypnotized into letting go. He wanted to let go of his fears, his annoyance at being kept awake by his wife's snoring, his discomfort with feeling suffocated. Instead he had wisely, but without conscious design, used his first sessions to lighten and unburden himself. Talking to someone who will not burden you in return can take a huge weight off your shoulders. Contrary to popular belief, therapy has often little to do with finding answers and even less with analyzing unconscious causalities. It has more to do with the primeval relief of finding oneself no longer alone.

Faith promises relief from the terrors of loneliness; love gives us an earthly taste. Listening to the plea of your sleep-deprived, tired self and saying: *I am right here, what can I do for you?* lightens the scariness of being alone as well. And that is something you can do for yourself.

This much is clear to me:

Finding something or someone to love almost invariably alleviates insomnia; Feeling abandoned, trapped, and alone almost always brings it on.

Have you been abandoning yourself? Do you feel trapped? If that's what happened, your sleep problems are a form of loss and grief. What you need to do is stop in your tracks; turn around and say:

Sorry! I didn't mean to forget all about you and leave you stranded. Do you need help?

CHAPTER 3
IN THE SPIRIT OF SLEEP

LAURA was one of my early workshop participants.

I owe her a lot of insight into the efficacy of sleep techniques—or the lack thereof. She had been a dancer in her younger years and now taught movement and theater at one of our local colleges. Laura was outspoken, efficient, and a longtime insomniac.

Usually I run my workshops for two evenings, one week apart. Laura gave me about one hour into the first evening before she spoke up. At the time I would have preferred if she had waited until after class; in retrospect, however, I came to appreciate her straightforwardness.

I am sorry, she interrupted, *but this is drivel. Your theories sound good but they don't work.*

I was flustered, and, I am sorry to say, not as kind as I would have wanted to be.

You are a teacher, Laura, I said, *you know that theories never work; it's people who do the work.*

I HAVE worked, believe me, Laura challenged me. *I know*

how to breathe, I am a yoga instructor; I know how to stretch, I went to EST seminars, remember EST? I know how to work with affirmations. I know how to apply myself, and I have. And nothing I do, no matter how well and how long I do it, brings me any closer to sleep.

The workshop had about fifteen participants; one was a man. He said that he had pretty much tried everything too but was still hopeful to learn something new.

These are the times when I wish I were a physician with a prescription pad and a new promising drug I could offer. My heart went out to these people who had come—some from out of state—in the hope of getting a break from their exhaustion.

On a scale from one to ten, I said—*ten being very upset and distressed, and one being pretty relaxed—where are you right now?*

People called out their numbers. There were a lot of sevens, some eights, one four. Laura was the last: *Ten,* she said reluctantly.

I am going to pace you through three minutes worth of breathing, I said. *If at all possible stay with me. I am going to count to eight or so for an exhalation, then to four for inhaling, then eight again for air out. Okay? We start on an exhalation. Ready?*

> *OUT: one, two, three, four, five, six, seven, eight*
> *IN: one, two, three, four*
> *OUT: one, two, three, four, five, six, seven, eight*
> *IN: one, two, three, four*

I WANT TO SLEEP

OUT: one two three, four five, six seven, eight, nine,
*   ten*
IN: one, two, three, four

We did this for about three minutes roughly sixteen cycles.

Thank you, I said to a noticeably calmer group. *On a scale from one to ten—same thing as before—how do you rate yourself?*

The numbers were considerably lower. They have to be. You can't breathe like that for several minutes and not calm down. Laura said she was between a six and a seven.

Now, please bear with me, I said: *One person gets up and stands behind a neighbor.*

I want pairs of one seated person and one standing behind them.

Right.

Now, put a hand on your partner's left shoulder—wait a second, there is more—and when you put that hand there, quietly say: "I am here, right behind you."

Go.

The room grew still.

Everyone take your seats again, please. We are doing another round of breathing. Then alternate partnering.

Quietly put your hand on your partner's shoulder and say:

"I am here, right behind you."

Let's do it.

Now, please take your writing pads and put your experience into words. Afterwards, if you want, we can compare notes.

You'd have to have been there, people say, when words seem inadequate. The room had grown quiet, heads were bowed; eyes stared unseeingly, accessing inner worlds.

After ten minutes or so—some people always write more than others—I said: *Please close your eyes.*

Now place your right hand on your left shoulder; in your mind say to yourself: "I am right here, I am behind you."

Tell me what happened.

This is a powerful exercise. It is based on the somewhat corny assumption that we all have a relationship with ourselves. Colloquially we refer to this relationship in sayings like: 'I had to have a talk with myself; "I let myself down", "she really didn't take care of herself."

This exercise makes the relationship explicit:You give yourself some air; then you announce your presence and your commitment.

Imagine doing this in the middle of the night when you are wide awake with worry. When you do that, you intentionally step in between the competing mind-sets "wired" and "tired". You literally give yourself a break, and now your insomnia can no longer escalate.

As an exercise, it IS an odd thing to do. Participating in it as part of a group makes it a little more palatable. One thing is certain, however. Deciding on this kind of breathing and affirming your supportive presence in real time will calm you down. And it will give you a break from internal scare tactics.

Laura called two days later to apologize for having been "abrupt". She also wanted me to know that she could not make the following workshop for employment reasons. I was sorry and missed her presence; so did the other group members.

I took it as a compliment when several women brought their husbands to the next and last session. Unfortunately that always plays havoc with the group dynamics and makes it difficult for the presenter to reactivate the original group spirit. Which poses an interesting question: Why are exercises less effective when the group process is interrupted? *It wasn't quite as good as last time,* people will say. Is there some kind of induction process that can't be skipped? A mood, a spirit that shouldn't be broken?

I believe there is. Good groups tend to bond and develop a version of team spirit over their lifetime.

We need a similar history in our nightly exposure to ourselves. That is especially crucial if our usual sleep dynamics are fraught with tension. Seeking ourselves out, *Zuwendung* works much more reliably once we have made it into a nightly ritual.

O sleep ... how have I frightened thee? Remember the Shakespeare quote? We have to know how to get into the spirit of sleeping, especially if our waking mood is overly dominant and had us leaning too far toward control and extraneous availability.

After all, sleeping is surrendering control and becoming available to internal necessities.

Setting the mood is a powerful resource. Sometimes the right mood is more important than the actual proceedings. The cooking more important than the eating. Anticipation more pleasurable than the actual trip. That is also true for sleep. Good sleepers get in the mood earlier in the evening. Not being in the mood can kill the best of intentions and trivialize the most elegant of techniques. Going to sleep is a highly mood-sensitive process and not just a matter of doing the right thing.

It was this realization that changed Laura's attitude toward sleep.

I always looked at sleeping as a performance, She said.

And being a performer, not being able to pull it off drove you crazy, I said.

Just about, said Laura.

And now that you see sleeping as a mood-related process?

That's an entirely different animal.

Laura was intense when she was on to something.

I WANT TO SLEEP

As a theater person, I know about moods. As a dancer I know about moods. You start setting it way before curtain time. It's a ritual thing, she said. *Lots of things have to be just right ...* Words failed her.

I think, I know, I said. *Good group process can set a mood. If that process is interrupted, the exact same presentation is less effective. That's what happened in the session you missed.*

How do you set the mood for sleeping? I asked; *I thought yoga and breathing was supposed to do that.*

Sorry about that little outburst, Laura said. *That wasn't* setting *the mood, that was* messing up *the mood.*

Laura, I said, *how could yoga and meditation possibly mess up the mood for sleeping? These techniques are documented to be effective; I know lots of people who swear by them.*

Everything and anything can mess up the mood, she said, *if it's done in the wrong spirit.*

These were very wise words indeed.

You can perform all the *right things* in the *wrong spirit,* and your body will know. Your lover will know, your baby will know, your pet will know.

The right sleep spirit is hearing your sleepless body's plea for your compassionate intervention: *If you love me, please ignore the wired mind activity and give me a hand with the tired.* Trying to trick your mind into sleeping when it wants to be in your comforting company is not the right spirit.

So, I said, *tell me how you evoke the sleep-mood spirit.*

Laura actually blushed. *I used to sleep in T-shirts, you know? Or my husband's pajamas? So, I bought myself this beautiful nightgown ...*

I thought I'd heard it all.

You have chronic sleep problems, and the cure is a nightgown? Can I quote you on that?

The nightgown is not the cure; of course not. Laura used her teacher's voice. *It's what goes with it; there is a whole setting that goes with it.*

A romantic setting? I asked.

No, yes, you could call it romantic; I am creating another world when I slip it on. It's a prop, if you want.

She closed her eyes, ever the theater person, *curtain,* she said, *and in my mind a play begins. It is fabulous. I can't wait to go to bed.*

You hated going to bed, I said.

I know, she said, *I am exaggerating; truth is I seem to be able to tell myself stories, act out whole scenes. There is a wonderful world going on behind my eyelids.*

Sometimes bad things happen behind people's eyelids, I said.

I WANT TO SLEEP

They would, and they could, Laura said. *That's where the playwright and the director come in.*

You are those too? I asked.

Definitely, Laura said. *It is a lot of fun; I never get to see the end, though.*

You fall asleep during the performance?

Night after night, Laura said.

And in costume too. (I couldn't help it.)

Sleep is not the only human function that defies things perfunctory and only thrives in the right spirit. There are lovemaking, child rearing, gardening, most artistic endeavors, even cooking. Without a loving, appreciative spirit, eating becomes calorie counting; work deteriorates into indenture, prayers into empty words, yoga into slimnastics, and sleeping into comatose checking out.

When Laura bought herself some fancy sleepwear, she drew on her sensitivities to mood and the right spirit. It was a playful, loving thing to do. Trivial, frivolous, maybe, but in the right spirit. Out of that creative commitment to the part that needed her most grew a whole new venture: nightly wonderful performances and in their wake, much-needed sleep.

COMMENTARY

Groups can set a mood, and a good facilitator will use this

spirit to further a group's process. As individuals we are usually not very skilled at modifying or even detecting our moods. Growing up has skewed our mood-spirit-inclinations with suspicions of "moodiness."

Laura's theater background gave her an advantage. The rest of us experience the power of spirit more by default. Have you ever had the misfortune of getting assigned to a team of competitive, ego-greedy people? Have you been in the company of well-meaning friends lately? Then you know that this kind of energy is something to reckon with.

Do you know how to make, invoke the difference?

It would be an invaluable skill to develop in the making of good nights. And not just good nights—days and relationships as well.

I grew up in a religious tradition called *Suebian Pietism.* It is steeped in rural spirituality, and I am sure that's why the Navaho invocation of a beautiful, good world speaks to me so powerfully. As I am talking about the importance of doing things in the right spirit—especially trying to get some sleep—it is only fair for you to ask: *And how do I do that, invoking the right spirit?*

There are gradations, a spectrum of sorts, when it comes to spirit. Setting a mood, creating an ambiance, getting in the swing of things are mundane invocations of spirit. Rituals, prayers, and sacred spaces are designed to help our minds switch from an ordinary state to a more spiritual one. Music is evocative on a nonverbal level, so are incense, rhythms, postures, and movements. All of that is to say that people always knew about the importance of states of mind and found ways to affirm their preferences. The right spirit is the right state of mind.

Even if you don't consider yourself a spiritual person, your state of mind is crucial for sleeping. Consider prayers. Prayers can alter our state of consciousness. That is especially true for prayers of gratitude and affirmation. For good sleeping a peaceful and beautiful world is the best of all worlds.

This is the world that traditional Diné (Navajos) invoke. Most are poor by our standards, life is hard, and their land is barren. Yet their faith affirms an abiding presence of beauty and harmony: Hózho.

Just imagine how much closer to sleep you could move by being of the same mind as these words. The prayer is an act of good will: THIS is the spirit I want to embrace and be embraced by. It is a treat.

Hózhóogo naasháa doo

In beauty I walk
With beauty before me I walk
With beauty behind me I walk
With beauty above me I walk
With beauty around me I walk

It has become beauty again
It has become beauty again
It has become beauty again
It has become beauty again

Hózhó náhásdlíí.

When you sleep you enter a world designed to heal. It is a way of living that is wondrously beautiful. When you enter there, living becomes sane again and the bruising realities of our waking-state are held at bay.

Another tradition, early Greek this time, also had a word for this sacred, protected space: *Temenos,* the blessed circle where broken things can mend again. Sleep, uncontaminated sleep, is such a beautiful mending place. Don't crash the circle. Honor it.

Adolescents are noted for their moodiness. They use music and clothes to set moods and get into the spirit in ways that many adults have lost. They can teach us something about the tremendous power of moods, good and bad, and the environments that create and support them. Unfortunately, they are often not their own playwrights nor their own directors.

CAROLINE

Caroline was accompanied by her mother.

She clearly did not want to be in my office, but her sleeping habits had deteriorated to such an extent that everyone was worried about her, parents and school alike. Her academics had slipped and absences accumulated. She fell asleep in class, and it was impossible to get her up in the morning. Her mom had bought several alarm clocks, and set them at staggered intervals. Caroline still had to be shaken awake, and verbally abused whoever had that onerous task. She missed the bus regularly and had to be driven to school—at great inconvenience to her family, who had their own schedules to keep.

They all do that, other mothers said; *it's the age.*

Only Caroline seemed to do more of it and was about to be suspended. It was either see a "shrink" or face serious consequences.

Caroline was seventeen and couldn't wait to get away and go to college.

At the rate you are going, Caroline, her mother said, *you won't be going to college at all.*

Caroline checked her messages.

Would you please not do that?

Her mother looked as if she had a migraine coming on. Caroline snapped her phone closed and gave me her prettiest smile.

Are you taking any medications, Caroline? I started.

Medications often work as mood-modifiers—with or without stated clinical indication. A chemically facilitated mental environment is hard to modify by psychological means. I also asked because over the past ten years 85 percent of my younger patients had been diagnosed and medicated for ADD or ADHD. Most of these medications are, technically speaking, stimulants and would make it hard for anyone to fall asleep at night.

I am not on the pill, if that's what you are asking.

Caroline's smile did not falter. Her mom gave her a shocked and me an embarrassed look.

Birth control pills can have a very stabilizing effect on women, I said, *but I was more thinking along the lines of Ritalin.*

I used to take that when I was younger, but I am not any more. She did an expert hair-fling. *It really messed with my brain big time, you know?*

You are not? Her mother's voice rose in alarm. She'd had no idea.

As I said, said Caroline.

How much sleep do you get?

Enough. Pretty much the same as everyone else.

Four hours? Six hours? Eight hours?

Eight hours? Caroline gave a dismissive snort. *I have a life, you know.*

Twelve hours when she has to spend time with her family, her mother said. *She pretty much slept through Christmas at her grandmother's.*

There was no reception in all of frigging New Hampshire. Caroline closed her eyes and shook her head incredulously.

Now Caroline, her mother said.

I WANT TO SLEEP

How much? I can be persistent.

I take naps, sleep on the bus. Four hours, maybe. All right?

You haven't taken a school bus in years, Caroline, please don't waste the doctors time, her mom said.

You're going to get sick on that little sleep, forget things, go on binges, I said.

Sleep and food have nothing to do with other, Caroline dismissed me.

Some people think they do, I said. *But sleep deprivation and obesity have definitely something to do with each other.*

She made a suspicious face. *What?!*

Big-time, I said. *Google it.*

I don't have insomnia, I keep telling her that. I can sleep at the drop of a hat.

But you don't, I said.

Not when I have better things to do, Caroline said.

Sleeping is magical, and you are missing out, I said.

Sleeping is for losers.

Then, after a minute or so, came the first little break:

My ex-boyfriend sleeps all the time, and he is a loser.

There are different ways to get away from unpleasant stuff, I said; *one is by oversleeping and the other by overwaking.*

There is no such word as overwaking, Caroline said.

It's when you are so ON all the time, so involved and plugged-in that you are too hyper to think and to feel much.

I think and feel plenty, Caroline said.

So, what do you think about graduating, and how do you feel about not having much of a future past high school?

I think and I feel plenty, Caroline repeated.

How much depth can there be to a person when they are flat-out? I asked.

Oh stop it, Caroline said and made a shoofly movement with her hand.

Caroline's mom had confided in me with some embarrassment that her daughter and her friends were Wiccans. I am sympathetic to people who wonder if life may not more of a web than a straight line. I sighed dramatically: *Sleep is magical. Compared to waking it is supernatural. Do you have any dreams, Caroline?*

I have plenty of dreams, she said.

Den seinen gibts der Herr im Schlaf, I said.

Caroline's parents insisted that the kids speak German at home—another major bone of contention.

I WANT TO SLEEP

They chose me partially because of my German background.

"Those who are the Lord's are being granted things in their sleep."

What is that supposed to mean? Caroline wrinkled her nose.

It is ancient wisdom, I said. *It means that there is a world of resources in our unconscious. We are smarter, wiser, and healthier in our sleep than we are when we are awake. All our mistakes are made when we are supposedly awake.*

She wore a Free Tibet button so I pulled all the stops: *You know what the Dalai Lama said?*

What?

"Sleeping is the best meditation."

I know all about the unconscious and dreams and stuff, Caroline said.

She had taken an elective in psychology, and wanted to be a psychologist. Maybe an animal psychologist.

Robby sleeps all the time, and believe me, he is not smarter or healthier than the rest of us.

Maybe sleeping keeps him out of trouble. I said. *Maybe he is depressed. Maybe he likes it better there. He does too much of it—you do too little. I can see why you were a couple. Opposites attract.*

Caroline gave me a hard stare. *He is depressed all right,* she said.

The second session a week later was rough. Caroline was alone because her mother had another doctor's appointment.

Do your parents have any idea how much pot you are smoking? I asked.

Caroline didn't even question how I knew.

It helps me relax.

Spoken like a true druggie, I said.

She just stared at me.

It's been almost a year now that Cindy died, right? I asked.

Caroline hugged a pillow and buried her face. About a year ago two local kids had been killed in a car accident. There had been four of them in a car going home from a party. The driver, Cindy, had not been drinking but lost control at high speed. In a small town the shock was palpable for months. The school initiated some "grief work" but a small group of girls took it upon themselves to hold nightly vigils on a knoll near the accident scene. I knew from some other kids that Caroline was most adamant about keeping the vigils alive. She also was the one supplying the pot.

You weren't in the car, right?

Caroline shook her head.

I WANT TO SLEEP

You weren't even that close friends, I understand.

I was supposed to go home with them, Caroline talked into the pillow.

My heart went out to her: two of her friends were dead and she was alive. It wasn't fair. Caroline's eyes behind the pillow were wide with dread: *I made them wait,* she whispered. *Finally they just left.*

And you think that's why Cindy was speeding .

Caroline just looked at me.

We don't know that, I said, *but one thing we know for sure.*

What? A muffled barely audible noise.

All four of them were talking at the same time. You can go fast, I said, *but not safely while you are yakking it up with your friends.*

After a long while, I said *Caroline?*

What?

You don't owe them. You deserve to have your life back.

I gotta go, Caroline said.

I did not expect Caroline or her parents to return for a follow-up appointment, yet they did. Caroline wanted to be dropped off; her mom would pick her up after the appointment.

Slouching in my couch she morphed from a young suburban sophisticate into a miserable girl. *I am suspended,* she said. *I fell asleep in English, and when Mr. Bates woke me up, and everybody laughed, I swore at him.*

And THAT got you suspended, I said.

I can't not graduate, Caroline wailed. *It'll ruin my life.*

You got in trouble because you are sleep deprived, I said. *That'll ruin your life. Sleep-deprived people make serious mistakes and eventually just crash. If you want to graduate, you have to get your act together really fast. You want me to tell you what to do?*

What?

Make a pact with your closest friends. From now until the end of the school year everybody HAS to sleep nine hours a night. Check up on each other, no excuses. And because this sounds uncool, keep it a secret.

Caroline was interested, kind of, and we spent the rest of the hour brainstorming logistics.

If they don't get it, can we all come and you tell them?

The kids did not come as a group.

I know from running into Caroline's mom at Stop & Shop, though, that she did indeed graduate. I don't know if Caroline and her friends formed a sleep pact. She is at college now; if I should happen to see her in town, I'll ask her.

I WANT TO SLEEP

COMMENTARY

My work with groups convinced me that setting the mood for trying something different is more effectively done when one is not the only one attempting it. I believe this to be especially true for reaching out to sleep, which is a lonely place to begin with. Women seem to be able to utilize this kind of group energy or group support more readily than men. Even male group members, however, were more willing to participate in exercises and rehearsals than they would have been in individual sessions. Group motivation also has a longer shelf life than individual efforts. There are, of course, also drawbacks and potential liabilities, which I will discuss in a later section of this book.

I did not see Caroline long enough to develop an alliance that would have neutralized her initial reluctance. Being dragged into counseling against your will never bodes well. I like to think though that my permission for her to return to the land of the living made a difference.

So here is what I *wish* I had done or could have done: Caroline lived in a neighboring town, and I knew the social service director there. She was a woman who worked toward her state license as a marriage and family therapist, and came to me for supervision. I could have asked her to give some thought to a sleep group, especially for high school seniors, and especially for girls. Maybe there could have been sleepovers—real sleep-dedicated nights at alternating houses.

Maybe the parents could have been sold on the idea. Maybe the parents also could have learned something about proper sleeping, about setting the right mood. Maybe I could have talked to them about sleep-conducive nutrition. Like solid breakfasts, light dinners, and no soft drinks or sweets during the day. Some warm milk and honey. Bedtime stories. Written summaries of the day: *what was your best moment?*

Maybe we could have talked about dreams.

KEVIN

Another person who was absolutely not in the mood for sleeping was Kevin. In many ways he could have been a friend of Caroline's.

Insomnia, I suggested earlier, could be seen and certainly used as an invitation to act as a soothing presence. What if something else already does that?

Kevin was fifteen, and described himself as a geek and a dork. He was a geek because he lived more in the virtual worlds of his computer than in real life—a differentiation that did not hold much significance for him any more. And he was a dork, because that's what he imagined girls saying about him.

Kevin had been an A-student until he got hooked on Second Life-type gaming. When I first saw him he looked disheveled and unkempt. His clothes were hanging from his body as if they'd been borrowed from someone two sizes larger. Kevin looked unhealthy and neglected, and he saw no reason whatsoever to be in any kind of therapy.

What was truly unusual about Kevin's situation was that both his parents came to the session with him. His mom, a local lawyer, and his dad, an insurance executive, were worried, as they had cause to be.

The referral had been made by the school social worker, who briefed me before the first appointment. She had known Kevin as a gangly, likable, witty kid, not much of an athlete unless you called skateboarding a school-approved sport. Everything looked as if Kevin would go far. He was the youngest of three. Both his brother and sister had left for college. One was due to graduate from Brown that spring. Then, about six months ago, things had begun to deteriorate at such a rapid rate that the school suspected drugs and called the parents in. Kevin was tested and came out negative. Next came physicals, and further blood work. Kevin was underweight but healthy. When grades began to slip further, truancies accumulated, and he was found sleeping in the bathroom, his parents were called in once more.

We established that Kevin was alone at the house most days, and if not alone then at least unsupervised. He had no friends he hung out with, and since this was winter, no real opportunity to go skateboarding. He claimed that he slept on weekends and declined to go snowboarding with his dad and older brother. Other than that his parents had to rely on the testimony of a Bolivian housekeeper who wished that Kevin would eat more but otherwise had no complaints, especially since he was the only one in the family who spoke passable Spanish.

Your parents and the school seem to think that you are severely sleep deprived, I told Kevin. *How much sleep do you get a night?*

Dunno, said Kevin without looking up.

How much time do you spend on the computer?

Couple of hours.

Eight hours? Ten hours? Twelve hours?

Kevin's head came up and he looked at me incredulously.

Twelve hours, no way! He said.

You mean to say that kids spend eight to twelve hours on the computer—a day? His father was flabbergasted.

They will and they do, I said. *Korea, the most wired country in the world, has huge problems with sleep-deprived teenagers who spend up to sixteen hours gaming until they collapse.*

I can't ... said his mother, at a loss for words.

We wouldn't know, Carol, Kevin's dad said.

Then to me*: Kevin took over his sister's apartment when she left for school. It is in an other part of the house.*

To make things worse, I said, *it's not just the amount of time Kevin spends staring at a screen; it is what overexposure to such an intensely limited focus does to his brain. He'll see text and images in his head for an hour after the screen goes blank, and couldn't sleep if he wanted to.*

Not an hour, Kevin said.

He had to put a supreme effort into not falling asleep in his chair. I had flashbacks of trying to stay awake in church on hot summer afternoons when I was a kid. It is an agonizing process, and more often than not a losing battle.

There was some irony in Kevin fighting to stay awake while most of my other clients fought to get some sleep.

What are we going to do? his mother said. *Kev, say something.*

Couldn't we just take him out of school for a couple of days and have him sleep it off? his father wanted to know.

It would be a start, I said. *You'd have to watch him, though, day and night. These games are highly addictive. He has pals waiting for him all over the globe. He'll be missed. Terrible things could happen while he is not in role.*

It's just a game, his dad said.

By now it is his whole life, I said.

Kevin had stopped participating and might as well have been asleep. We let him be, while I gave his parents their assignments:

- Restrict access to all computers in the house, and inform the school to do the same.
- Check his computer and see what he is involved in. If you can't access it, get someone who can.
- Read up on gaming. Google it, go to a bulletin

board and see if there is a support group for addicts or parents of addicts in your general area.

- Have him sleep on a cot in your room until we have a plan in place.

Kevin's parents were numb. They had expected some serious heart-to-heart, not a hard-core intervention for their teenaged addict.

Very luckily for Kevin, his family pulled together. He could not have broken free alone, even if he wanted to, and would eventually have ended up in a hospital. His sister, a budding software developer, came down from Boston and verified what we had suspected. Kevin was gaming most nights until daybreak.

When he was denied access to a computer, he went berserk and physically attacked his sister. Then he broke down crying. Then he ran away. The parents of an old buddy, where he showed up after twelve harrowing hours, brought him back home. He looked like a broken prisoner, his dad told me. He had not eaten, or showered, and had slept in someone's freezing garage.

It was his father who took a leave of absence and stayed home with him.

This is what needs to happen, Kevin, I said at our next planning meeting.

I can only help you with recalibrating your sleeping. For the gaming addiction you need other help.

110

I WANT TO SLEEP

You stay in your parents' bedroom. This can be done in the course of a week or so. Every night you lie down at eleven. No naps during the day. If you sleep, fine, but you have to get up at six every morning. If you don't fall asleep at night after half an hour, you get up and play chess or something with your dad. For another half hour. Then everybody goes back to bed. If you sleep, fine. If you don't, it's half an hour tossing and turning, then half an hour up with some activity in an other room. Your parents will help you make that happen. Same routine all night—every night until six in the morning. Then everybody gets up, has breakfast, and maybe your dad will do something with you all day long. I don't care what you do as long as it isn't sleeping or gaming.

It was a grueling week for everyone involved. When I saw them three days later for a checkup, it was hard to tell who was more exhausted, Kevin or his dad. Kevin had slept the first nights but still couldn't stay awake during the day. Then somehow the pattern reversed and he couldn't go to sleep at night and was wired during the day as well. He was an emotional mess and unbearable to live with. On their own, the family realized that watching TV was probably not a good idea either. If Kevin couldn't sit in front of a screen, nobody could. Their lives were turned upside-down.

Toward the end of the week mom helped out; over the weekend his brother and sister took care of him.

These are the very bare bones of sBMT: sleep-related behavior modification therapy.

Very few people are as blessed as Kevin was and is. His family was there for him in a way that is uncommon in my experience. It was inspirational, and, I believe surprised even them.

After ten days of basic BMT, Kevin slept through the night and functioned during the day. We then gave him an extra two hours, so he had now nine hours of night sleep. Then he went back to school. Computers were off limits for another month, and the school knew not to let him near one.

One of the core concepts of systemic therapy is that troubled individuals are often mere symptom-bearers. They are being identified as the only sick ones while the larger system, Kevin's family for example, was in danger of falling apart.

Kevin had been somewhat of an afterthought in family planning. When the older kids had flown the nest both parents resumed their professional careers, glad for Kevin's low-maintenance style. He seemed fine on his own, which was a relief for parents with demanding careers.

I think, it is fair to say that in the end Kevin kept his family together and saved his parents' marriage. Not long after his recovery they came to me for marital therapy. Their relationship had suffered from decades of neglect. For most of their married life, all emotional resources—in terms of time and priorities—had been devoted to the kids. Kevin's dad especially felt deprived of emotional connectedness. He had been the breadwinner for most of the earlier years—years that he described as professionally rewarding but emotionally barren.

In a letter, Kevin's older sister thanked me for my role and wistfully added: *I know it might sound weird to you, but I am envious of the time Kevin got to spend with my dad.*

It did not sound weird to me. It was sad.

COMMENTARY

Kevin did not get enough sleep, but he would never have described himself as an insomniac. Yet he shared an insomniac's difficulty with minimizing overload and engaging in self-soothing. Instead of spending time on agonizing adolescent self-doubts he immersed himself in a virtual world—an escape that could have cost him dearly. This immersion in a world of his own might sound crazy to people of a different vintage, but it is not that much more of an artifact than many corporate cultures, and just as exclusive, arcane, and addictive. I wondered if Kevin's dad did not have an inkling of those faint parallels when he decided to stay home with his boy in a move so uncharacteristic that it shocked everyone who knew the family. Virtual realities of any kind can have significant emotional rewards. They can make a person feel connected, important, validated, and alive. But they are the psychological equivalents of junk food—tasty but ultimately unhealthy. Unhealthy because virtual almost always means collapsed timing and suspended accountability. Messing with our sense of timing is as disorienting as being in a wrong place, and lack of consequences precludes real learning. A body and mind that have been synchronized to virtual realities fall out of step with the much slower and much more complex rhythms of organic life. Choices without real-life consequences stunt emotional intelligence. When that happens, life as we know it becomes boring and delays in gratification are met with impatience and physical intolerance. People interrupt each other impatiently, one month is a long-term relationship, and a five minute delay can lead to road rage. *Waiting* becomes a bad word and a bad thing, and making insightful connections seems beyond reach. Waiting for sleep too becomes an imposition, and the link between bad days and bad nights is no longer self-evident.

There are developmental theories that directly link a person's ability to wait (delay of gratification) to maturational levels. Kevin at one time joked that he would have slept more if he only could have slept *faster*. A lot of people who come to see me are impatient with their sleeping. They are convinced that they have more important things to do, and sleeping, especially *waiting* for sleep, makes them edgy and angry.

Sleep, on the other hand, has all the time in the world.

Kevin responded to behavior modification therapy not only because of the efficacy of this approach but especially because his family closed ranks around him, a concept that translated into spending lots of time with him. This kind of reprogramming is rigorous and demanding. Few patients succeed at it without sustained, loving support from caring people.

CHAPTER 4
WHEN WAKING AND SLEEPING
BECOME INDISTINCT

There is a voiceless minority in our midst that has no economic or political clout. They might as well, as Mary Pipher calls it, live *in another land.* These are our elderly parents, relatives, former neighbors, and friends. Older people are by and large lonely, often medicated, and physically uncomfortable, depressed, and without life's hope of a better tomorrow. They often have lost their lifelong mates and childhood friends; their homes; their professional status; their good looks and physical fitness; their financial independence; their hearing, eyesight, and sense of taste. The rest of the world has a hard time dealing with them because we can't tolerate the predictability of our own impending old age.

This has not been true for all societies at all times. No longer having to procreate or make a living afforded unprecedented artistic and philosophical freedom, and being the custodians of decades worth of skills and knowledge imparted importance and dignity. In our own society, though, when we assess a person's value, we mean their net worth. We rarely appreciate anyone anymore for their contribution to the quality of our lives. Women who brought up children and cared for grandchildren retain real and felt value almost independent of age. Men who traditionally served only auxiliary roles in nurturing and sustaining the next generation experience a loss of meaning and personal relevance that, I believe, accelerates their demise. Unless they stay active and involved, their life expectancy is noticeably lower than that of women.

STAN

Ron, an old friend from college days, was worried about his dad, who lives in an upscale retirement community nearby. He asked me to visit his father, who complained regularly about lying awake all night.

Stan had been a farmer all his life, and made good financially when he sold most of his fertile river land to a mall developer. That was over twenty years ago, and Stan was still ambivalent about having sold land when I met him.

Having grown up in a farming community, I knew the value of land. You didn't ever sell land unless you absolutely had to. Land would be handed down through generations, and selling it was tantamount to robbing your kids and grandchildren of their livelihood and future. The land fed you, housed you, protected you, gave you roots, meaning, and continuity, and kept you humble. Without land you lost your freedom, your standing, your way of life—*everything.*

Nobody wanted to work the farm anymore, Stan told me. *You want them to get an education and do better than their parents and grandparents and next thing you know they can't be bothered working with their hands no more.*

My people had worked their land for hundreds of recorded years, I said, *then the same thing happened.*

My people were dirt-poor when they came from Poland, Stan said. *Do you know what dirt-poor means?* He told me anyway. *They were so poor they didn't even own no dirt. Then they came here into the Valley and got themselves some of the best farming land in the whole United States. Excepting the river flooding occasionally you can grow anything here, sell it to Boston, and still have enough. When I was a kid I remember going down to Boston in a rattletrap of an old truck delivering wholesale. Four hours each way. That was in addition to working the farm. I was maybe ten or twelve at the most.*

Stan had met me in the lobby and started the conversation with: *I don't mean no disrespect, but I don't need no head doctor.*

I had smiled. *The longer I look around the more I think EVERYBODY needs a head doctor.*

You got a point there, Stan agreed.

Can you walk? I asked. *It's a sin sitting inside on a day like this.*

The way Stan took in the weather, the shrubs, and the endangered dandelions on the classy lawn reminded me of my grandfather. It is the look of a craftsperson handling a piece of wood, or the look of a good mechanic listening to a troubled engine. This was his world out here. He knew

117

the tell-tale signs, the smells, the nuances, and the significance of every event.

This lawn here, he said, *is crap. It is a waste of good land, waste of water, and the fertilizer pollutes the ground, kills them worms, and with it the birds that eat them. I hate seeing it, I really do.*

And I bet the activities people want you to take leisurely strolls and enjoy all the beautiful landscaping your money buys, I ventured.

Stan leaned on his walker. *If it weren't for you, I'd go back in.*

I felt a wave of sadness rolling in on me. "Inside" for a farmer is like being hog-tied; idle, useless. Outside for Stan was a reminder of what he had lost.

Are they composting? I asked.

Yes, they do, Stan said. *Let me show you.*

Composting has always fascinated me. Not only because it makes such good soil but for almost spiritual reasons. Where else do you come face to face with nature's forgiving, non-judgmental ways: Out of garbage and refuse, yucky stuff we don't even want to touch, microorganisms, sunlight, worms, and rain make the best growth medium money could ever hope to buy. Good coming out of bad. Another kind of wisdom. Amazing grace.

What do you think, I said, *what makes better compost,*

people's buried bodies, or just their ashes?

Bodies, but it takes longer; Stan said, not in the least put out. Not even surprised—*When I was in my early twenties, what would be my father-in-law who was horse-crazy, had a mare die on him. He dug a hole—this was before dozers, mind you—and buried her. Many years later, the grass was still greener there and the apples he planted bloomed earlier.*

That makes a good story, I said.

Yeah, Stan laughed and spit on a pile of last fall's leaves. *Right. I tell it to the social worker and she tells the nurse, and before you know it I have a new pill in my little pink tray.*

Pink, I said, *they make you eat things off pink trays?*

You come back, Stan said.

I will; I promised Ron we'll talk about your sleeping.

Stan was much less alert when I visited him a week later. It was raining and we couldn't visit the compost pile. I expressed regret, but Stan said:

The rain is good. We need it this time of year. Soaks the roots, you know.

You know what the Indians call it? I asked.

What?

This kind of light and steady rain, they call it "she-rain."

Makes sense, Stan said.

He was staring straight ahead:

Sometimes, you know ... He looked up at me to make sure I was with him; so many of his buddies were no longer "with it" or if they were they couldn't hear much. *Sometimes I don't rightly know if I am awake or if I'm sleeping. It's all blending together, like. I don't know if maybe I just dreamt something, you know? Or if it really happened.*

Does that bother you? I asked. *Do you mind?*

I do and I don't.

He thought a minute, then said:

I do because I don't want to waste precious time; being I don't have much left. And I don't because it doesn't make a damned difference anyway.

Some of it could be the medications, I said. *I'll have Ronnie checking it out for you.*

That would be good, Stan said.

I have been thinking about that compost pile, I said. *How it makes black gold out of waste.*

Gotta pee, Stan said.

When he got back he said: *I talked to Ronnie the other day, and he said I should listen to you because you have a way with words.*

If you are up for it, I said.

I am up for it, Stan said. *God knows I have nothing better to do.*

Can you still write? I asked.

Barely, he said *but I have a laptop somewhere.*

He grinned broadly at my surprise. *Used it on the farm in the last years—a spare one from Sophie my grand-daughter—one of them.*

Laptops or granddaughters? I said

Funny, Stan said after a moment—*should've been a Comedian.*

About the writing, I said, *it's going to be titled:*

'STAN'S COMPOST PILE'

Stan nodded. He knew exactly where this was headed.

All the bad stuff, the unmentionables, the unacceptable, the objectionable, the offensive, even. All the waste of life.

Like my being an alcoholic? Stan said.

Ronnie didn't say anything about that, I said.

Hell, I never said anything about that, Stan said. *Nobody ever said anything about it.*

Write it down, I said. *Put it on a paper pile; see what time and life's tossing and turning did with it. How it got composted. Everything does get eventually composted, barring plastic bottles. black gold—at the very bottom of the pile is where the black gold is. See what came out of it.*

What do you mean, black gold? I sold the black gold to the mall guys, Stan said. *Got myself some real gold instead. And lookee here what it bought me.*

There was pain in his voice.

A callused hand reached for mine. *Sorry, I didn't mean that.*

Stan had surprisingly little trouble writing. Part of it was, I guess, that he had no expectations. Stan wrote his heart out. The staff told me that he sat at his table several hours in the early mornings and on and off during the day. He didn't offer for me to read his material, and I didn't ask to see it. The "composting" was a private matter.

Stan's readiness and fervor to write pleased and concerned me. Things are usually not that easy. What if he hit a snag beyond just writer's block? What if he revisited some serious traumatic events that refused to be appropriated by the composting metaphor? What if he precipitated a depression by digging around in his past? He *was* depressed when I'd met him first.

I asked him.

I WANT TO SLEEP

I have regrets, sure I do; I have more regrets than things to be proud of.

Do they keep you up? Does that get you down?

You know, he said, *there is one thing about having farmed all your life long: You make all kinds of decisions, but what comes of it is up to the weather. My wife she used to tell me all the time: "Stan you should've; Stan you shouldn't have" It drove me crazy.*

People do stupid things, I said. *I don't mean your wife...*

I know what you mean; But when your horse kicks you, whose fault is that? When I tried to lift some equipment off my neighbor's foot and popped a hernia—stupid, right? But whose fault was it? When you end up working a couple of wet acres or start hitting ledge, there's no point getting depressed. When you got hay sitting out there and it rains, are you gonna blame yourself? Should'a got it done yesterday?

But, I said, clearly losing my therapeutic edge, *but people have choices and ...*

Choices my ass, Stan said. *People ain't better than animals and sometimes not even smarter, and they can't help it if they are made up one way or the other. You are at the mercy of things when you farm, you know?*

Well, I thought to myself *there goes my whole rationale for being a therapist.*

You came to ask about my sleeping, right? Stan changed

the subject.

I didn't have to worry about him being depressed.

How is your sleeping?

When I sleep, I sleep; he said. *When I'm awake, I'm awake. I like it either way. I am always pondering what I write, though. Dream about it too.*

When it was time to go he shook my hand good-bye: *Don't worry about me; I'm good.*

If only we all could say that.

The staff told me that Stan was rarely napping during the day and had not asked for "something to sleep" in weeks. He also seemed to move around with more coordination. He changed from an ornery old man—old women are so much easier to care for the aides told me—to a witty old man.

Only once did Stan get bent out of shape. A young aide asked him if he'd backed his stuff up. After clarifying a physiological misunderstanding, he panicked.

You mean all I've written could just disappear?

Stan typed with two arthritic fingers, he told me. He worked very hard as he always had; the thought off all his labor having been for naught must have cut to the bone. He lost the farm—or sold it, which to him was all the same; this book of his was his last attempt at leaving a legacy. You worked hard, put your heart and soul into it and then let nature take care of the rest. I envied him for his lack of hesitation. Stan understood what he was doing even though the terms *symbolic* or *metaphorical* would have meant nothing to him.

Fortunately the aide was not only sensitive; she also knew what to do. Two hours later Stan's life was saved on disk.

Lindsay, the young woman, gave him another huge gift. Without quite knowing what she had done to deserve Stan's gratitude, she told me about showing him how to use the spell-checker. Like many others whom I have encouraged to become tellers of their story, Stan was mortified about his spelling.

The staff was proud to have a writer among their residents and wanted to know how many pages he had written on any given day.

Stan was busy with an urgency almost unbecoming to a barely ambulatory octogenarian.

When he died unexpectedly six months later; he had written over three hundred pages of his life's stories. It was a gift, Ronnie told me, more precious than all the Wal-Mart-money. Like a good farmer, I couldn't help but thinking, he had waited until fall to take his final rest.

COMMENTARY

Many times during my work with people who can't sleep, I have noticed the same phenomenon: When something important happened, insomnia became less important.

Sleep duration might still be curtailed, but it was no longer an all-consuming issue. By important I mean Stan getting his life "composted"; Kevin and his dad shopping and cooking together for the family, Lydia helping to deliver a breech. Girls tapping into their collective power. Cheryl taking pleasure in engaging her mind in her own behalf.

It is difficult to home in on that personal, real importance, for therapists and patients alike. Somehow we don't seem to know what it is before we come upon it. It doesn't call attention to itself the way other important things do: getting medical attention, taking advantage of the stock market. Quiet time, though—oftentimes quiet times at night—seem to make that importance stick out a bit more. Maybe the retreat of other voices makes it more audible.

Sometimes I found, the thing-of-importance isn't a thing at all, it can be a direction. Sometimes it is a return to an old love. At any rate, when you can't sleep it might be wise to be on the outlook for what's quietly calling attention to itself.

In your writing you could ask: *I don't know anymore what's really important. Do you?*

You mean important to YOU?

Of course I mean important to me. To whom else?

I haven't thought about it.

Think about it, then.

I know what USED to be important to me, us; does

that count?

It's a start.

Sleeping, of course, is important too; but when you get that unbidden extra thinking time, why not use it to find out what would fill your heart?

Even just realizing that it is your heart that needs filling is a huge step in the right direction.
A laurel fit to rest on.

CHAPTER 5
SUMMARY

But you have no need to go anywhere;
Journey within yourself.
Enter a mine of rubies
And bathe in the splendor of your own light.

Rumi

The stories I told you were—in a way—lost-and-found stories. As people explored their loss of sleep they found that they had lost much more. Stan had lost his usefulness; Kevin his family; Lydia lost her purpose, and Allan his freedom. As they reached out to their longed-for sleep, they reached out to themselves. From being at odds with themselves, they became agents in their own behalf. When I asked, *What do you think is the most important thing you learned,* there was a common denominator. Cheryl—I think—expressed it the best: *Even before I had these horrendous sleep problems, I was always afraid. Working with my insomnia taught me the difference between being scared and scaring myself. I always thought being scared was just my personality. When I started monitoring what was happening at night I realized that I was doing the scaring to myself; and I began to see HOW I did it too.*

This is a vastly important discovery. Once she saw that, she could intervene and make things intentionally better for herself.

But they found more than just an insight and a skill. Cheryl found an ally in herself, a new job, and incidentally also a new relationship. Laura found a way to make the magic of theater work for her and not just for her audience. The young women found a way to turn their collective power into an asset, and Kevin found a place in his own family— something he had never had before.

You too might have to find out the difference between being upset and upsetting yourself, a difference that affects more than just your bad nights. But even beyond that, I think it would be wise to look farther than insomnia. Ask yourself: *What have I lost?* I bet there will be more missing than just a sleep skill or even sleep itself. Spend time on understanding yourself. Be patient. If there is no time during the day, an hour at night can be a gift and a blessing.

Here is a bare-bones **summary of the techniques** employed in the preceding cases. But please keep in mind: Techniques are dry and lifeless by themselves. Sometimes they come across as outright corny. Imagine for example telling a fighting couple: *It is important that you start listening to each other.* Or, for that matter, imagine telling a wide-awake insomniac: *Why don't you relax and take a few deep breaths?* Bordering on the trivial, right? Yet as a technique listening skills are unsurpassed, and breathing exercises are absolutely essential. Many people and therapists-in-training love techniques. So, here they are. If you are in your right mind sleep-wise, they can become valuable tools.

Without it they end up just being one more tedious thing to try.

So, be aware of the spirit. Ask, *What can I do for you?* If you listen carefully—more often than not—you will hear: *Don't scare me, please.* Embrace your tired self, lovingly. Let the warm spirit of your *"Zuwendung"* make your eyes smile. And: Don't rush!

- *For paying attention and tuning in*

  Always start with making time to breathe. Make an extra effort to exhale so you'll have enough room for fresh air. Instead of *taking* a breath, *give* one. *Giving a breath*—a very long exhalation—has an unintended side effect: It makes you feel grateful for the air you get to inhale right after. *Gratefulness* is the name for a wonderful mental drug. Treat your self. There is nothing like it to counteract the sorry feelings that make for so many bad nights. Use your insomnia to appreciate these subtleties.

  Progressive relaxation of tense muscles is another way to tune into your physical self. For more information consult the workbook section. Start keeping a sleep book right away. A sleep book is a journal for your nightly musings; writing things down affords them a higher degree of reality than just thinking. You want positive experiences, not just positive thoughts.

- *For listening and letting go of distracting, pressing business*

Start practicing during the day. Start with VERY small steps:

> Ask: *How much of what is going on is scary and how much is me scaring myself?* Listen to the difference. Expose your mind to *waiting.* Feel the mental work that is involved in exercising patience. Breathe when your stomach gets antsy.

> For just plain listening, try to repeat—verbatim—the last two sentences your spouse just said to you. Make a game out of it and switch sides when you got a 100 percent endorsement:
> *Yes! That's exactly what I said.*
> Or imagine the insights you might gain from this simple writing/listening exercise: on top of your page write *What do you want me to pretend?* Then start listing what comes to mind. Pretending is expensive. Feel the price.

> Practice the soft-eye exercise suggested in the workbook section.

> Practice letting go exercises from the workbook.

- *For staying focused*

Start with staying with your breathing for ten cycles.

> Count: OUT one, two, three, four, five,

six, seven, eight
IN one, two,
OUT one, two, three, four, five, six,
seven, eight

- *For curbing your judgmental impulses*

Start by not voicing them. Practice *not* saying
things that are on the tip of your tongue. Notice
how pushing your opinions onto others almost
never works anyway. You always have a choice
in interpersonal exchanges. You can:
express support,
show curiosity, or
show disapproval.

Judgment comes when we don't approve.
Experiment with choosing curiosity instead.
How did you arrive at this decision?
What prompted you to ...?
Help me understand.

Write your journal until the internal editor goes
off-line and your words flow unthinkingly. For
detailed instructions and encouragement, read
Julia Cameron's book *The Right to Write.*

- *For becoming a soothing presence*

Notice how you scare yourself—and decide
against it. Comfort yourself instead.

Talk to children, especially when they are
unhappy. Know and feel the power of basic

soothing words like:

> *I am here for you.*
> *I love you.*
> *You are doing the best you can.*
> *You can count on me.*

Say those words every chance you get. First to others; it seems less odd. Then to yourself.

- *For inviting confidences*

Confide. Maybe confide in a therapist first, then in a trusted friend. Honor the courage it takes. Become a safe person: never betray a confidence. If you invite someone (or yourself) to freely speak their mind, never use that information against them. Insomnia is a lonely place to be. So is having secrets. In your writing—especially your initial nightly writing– say:

> *This is something I never told anyone.*
> *This is something I never said aloud.*
> *This is something I hate to even think about.*

Write it down—then make sure it remains confidential even if that means your notes have to be destroyed.

CHAPTER 6
THE ROAD AHEAD

I nsomnia research is in its infancy, and often focuses on specific biochemical aspects.

This book is less about insomnia and more about what you can do to get back on good terms with sleep. If that is what you want to do, there is a lot of rethinking ahead of you and many little changes that need to be made. For that reason, it is a good thing to keep in mind what we all know instinctively: We learn mostly from our mistakes, and we learn more effectively in groups.

SLEEP GROUPS

Imagine how sustaining and encouraging it would be to hear others talk about their own victories and defeats, their mistakes and their hard earned insights. Group support is a powerful tool: We are not alone; we are not the only ones. We can lean on each other, laugh at and with each other. Some things simply can't be sustained by going it alone. Having companions on the road to sleep is a wonderful gift. Look around you; how many sleep-deprived people do you personally know? How many resources can you count on? The vast majority of medical attention is given to sleep apnea. You need someone who understands insomnia—what it takes to get the sleep you want.

I want to encourage you to send out invitations to form a *sleep group*.

Almost everyone you talk to will admit to occasional or even severe problems with sleeping. Most of your friends use prescription drugs intermittently to fall asleep, and many of them will admit to uneasiness about becoming too dependent on them. Get together. Imagine discussing parts of this book together. Imagine being able to elaborate on what works, makes sense, or does not fit. Imagine being able to go over exercises with a supportive, reliable group of people who know exactly what you are going through. Imagine setting some small goals until you meet again. In the meantime do selected exercises for two weeks in a row, and check in with each other when daunting sleep challenges loom ahead.

There is no doubt that being part of a sleep group can significantly enhance the benefits you hoped for when you started reading this book.

Groups, though, have a life of their own, and some dynamics are predictable.

Small groups tend to deteriorate faster, because one or two absentees render the meeting mute. Remember how the group spirit suffers when the group composition changes? Make a commitment to your sleep group. There is also a constant inclination toward socializing—especially if the host provides snacks. You can counteract these dynamics by being aware of them and sticking to a vision statement.

Every group goes down this road. It is not your or someone else's fault. Have a manifesto, a vision statement:
This is what we want to do.
This is what we're trying to avoid.

Larger groups tend to split into sub groups that chat independently; troubled group members dominate or rarely participate. If you can't sit in a circle, the group is too big.

It might be a good initial practice to designate a leader to keep the group on track. Ask every second meeting or so: *How is The Group doing?* This is a special-purpose group, and you did not intend it to be yet another social gathering.

There is also a more sleep-specific reason to proceed with determination. Purposefulness, and a sense of accomplishment feel good, and feeling successful in any measure reinforces progress and helps you sleep more easily.

Here are some guidelines for keeping your group valuable and alive.

- Try to assure a membership of around eight people; more members tend to split the group, fewer leave holes if someone can't make it.
- Have a stated agenda.
- Call the group to order. Have a fixed date; start on time; agree on the next meeting right in the beginning.
- Allow for special needs or celebrations, then follow a previously agreed-on curriculum.
- Spend at least 30 percent of your group time writing. Writing is more introspective even if it is later shared. Talking triggers social

conventionalities, and interpersonal dynamics, and can be more agitating than calming. Some people rarely speak; others are unstoppable. Writing is a great leveler.

- Agree on homework, and encourage accountability.
- Inform the group if your plans or intentions have changed; waiting around for someone who might still be coming is hard on the nerves, and destructive to the group.
- Predictability, and small successive steps are calming and reassuring.
- Be vigilant about keeping the focus on the spirit of reaching out to sleep and not just on anti-insomnia technology.

SLEEP RETREATS

Sleep retreats are weekends or weeklong dedicated commitments.

I would like to see spas or inns offer them not only as economically viable alternatives to physical respites, but also as a public service.

Women especially, and most especially young mothers, need to get away to reset their sleep habits.

These retreats should be planned and facilitated by a professional; then carefully coordinated with the manager and especially the chef. There are indicators that certain food groups, and certainly the timing of the meals, can aid better sleeping.

Tryptophane-rich foods can serve as precursors to increased serotonin production, which in turn has been linked to enhanced metabolic stress management and easier sleeping. Nutritional sleep enhancements still suffer from hype and insufficient research. We know much more about what does NOT work, and menus need to take this into account. Caffeine, for instance, ingested early in the morning, may still act as a stimulant by bedtime.

The retreat leader should be trained as an individual and group therapist, because withdrawal from stimulus overload or chemical stimulants destabilizes us emotionally before it yields the peace of mind we hope for.

Medical backup should be available, and allowances made for participants with specific pharmacological needs.

It is my belief that extensive writing should be part of the curriculum. People comfortable with poetry and the magical, mind-frame-changing use of words should be encouraged to share their skill, and read to the group at bedtime.

Facilities and climate permitting, allowances should be made to sleep in the open air.

Sleep-adverse, self-important egos who have a hard time surrendering control, tend to reduce in size under a star filled sky. There is nothing like it to put our troubles in better perspective.

SIEGFRIED HAUG

O sleep! O gentle sleep!
Nature's soft nurse,
How have I frightened thee?
That thou no more
Wilt weigh my eyelids down
And steep my senses
In forgetfulness?

William Shakespeare,
Henry IV, Part 2

Though hast frightened yourself
And run away
From where your healing lies.
Come, soothe yourself
As a good friend would do
And speak of comfort
To your tired needs.

Siegfried Haug

CHAPTER 7
WORKBOOK

Act without doing;
Work without effort.
Accomplish the great task
By a series of small acts.

Tao Te Ching

Therapy, in my experience, is unpredictable. I know we are supposed to have treatment plans, set goals, list interventions, and tell the HMOs when we'll be done with it. In real life, however, therapy is concentrated living, and as full of surprises as any of our days. The stories in this book give you a taste of how nonlinear unlearning insomnia can be. Your own sleep story will, in all likelihood, have just as many twists and turns. Know that this is how it is supposed to be. Think of yourself as a growing tree: branches in all directions, leaves in season, more roots than you can imagine. Everything BUT straight and linear progress. If you need to measure your progress, don't do it by how much faster you can fall asleep. Do it by noting how much more time you have spent getting to know yourself. Do it by differentiating between *being worried* and *worrying yourself*; being upset and upsetting yourself. How fast can you catch on? Notice how waking up a couple of times is no longer a big deal.

Use the following exercises as you feel moved and as you see fit. Pick and choose. But first have a little dialogue with yourself:

I know I should do some of these exercises.

   So why not do them?

They are hokey. Plus I don't like exercising.

   So how do you plan on putting this book to use?

I hoped it would just kind of rub off on me.

   Dream on, buddy.

You know what would really be a good thing? Find someone to do the exercises with. Make dates and read to each other what came to mind. Do each other's lists.

A text, like this book, can make useful suggestions and put you on the road. But real learning comes from making mistakes. You can't learn from your mistakes by reading a book—only a live context will make you wise to that.

Exercises are the equivalent of a hands-on experience. There is a vast difference between knowing how to change a tire and changing a tire, knowing all about kids and being a parent. **At night you need to be experienced and not just knowledgeable**. So practice.

Let's start with Stan's story; nature's way of composting

fertile soil from otherwise appalling stuff. Such as insomnia.

Insomnia opened the door for Kevin and his dad to spend time with each other. It afforded an opportunity for writing or bird-watching. Sleeplessness could be a wake-up call as it was for Sheryl or Allan; or a teaching: *Mind the spirit, not just your technique;* something Laura came to appreciate.

The following exercise can tweak your mind into looking at things from a new perspective.

Write on a piece of paper:

> *My greatest strength can be my biggest weakness;*
> *My greatest weakness can be my biggest strength.*

Every night, for a week, list five areas of your life where you found this to be true. This is a non specific exercise and will not cure your insomnia—but it might set the stage. Your sleep problems too might have unappreciated dimensions.

You need to know.

PRACTICING BASIC REQUIREMENTS

Insomnia gives you a chance to spend time with yourself. This time can be either pure hell or it can be the beginning of a highly rewarding relationship. Few things are as beneficial to sleeping as caring relationships. They all have basic ingredients.

- They thrive if you know how to be present.
- You have to know how to put preoccupations aside so you can listen.
- You have to know how to be a soothing presence and avoid intimidation.

When you are suffering from insomnia you are preoccupied. You are not present.

FIRST AID

The following exercises are for the middle of the night.

(If you practice them during the day, proficiency will improve.)

To become present to your own body/self, first focus on **breathing.**

Count to 12 on an exhalation.
To 2 as you inhale.
Use your fingers to count off 10 sequences.

If you have been tossing and turning, make sure you are fully awake; only then can you take the lead.

Next, **relax your muscles** by tensing them up first. Use muscles that are unlikely to cramp. Your shoulders, your facial muscles, your hands.

I WANT TO SLEEP

Make a fist, and tighten one arm.
Hold tight while you count to 20 or until your
muscles start quivering.
Now: drop your arm and let go.
This is how relaxation *feels*.
Do it with other parts of your body.

You are now present and awake enough to **listen** to
yourself.

Turn on your light and get a hold of your sleep book.
You do have sleep book, right?

Have you been using scare tactics on yourself?
List them.
Which ones are old standbys? Notice your
clichés and generalizations. There will be plenty
of those.

List 15 things that would have been sleep-
friendly, sleep-conducive things to do today,
if you had only thought of them. Start with
getting up and end with going to bed.

These are things that you could, maybe,
consider doing tomorrow.

Now:
Use a stack of sticky notes and compile a list of
troublesome, intrusive concerns.
One per note.
Write on the sticky side.
Post them all around you on your bed sheet.
Try to be exhaustive.

Now:
One by one read them, then fold them, and seal
the ends.
Carefully place your paper loops by your night
table.
For tonight, that's where they'll stay.
We are not advocating denial.
You only put them aside for NOW.

You have now made room for a **visit.**

Say these words to yourself, whisper them if
necessary:

Hi, I am right here.
I am right here with you.
I don't want to scare you.

Now
Say back to yourself,
There is something I need to tell you.
- Say a secret, something difficult to
  admit—even to yourself.
- Breathe for yourself.
- Maybe write some of it down.

Now:
Tell yourself a story.
Make it a delightful, magical, unlikely story full
of delicious gratifications.
You know what they are.
Imagine magical powers that soothe your
worries.
Tomorrow you'll tackle them, ready and rested.

Tonight you make them go away so you can sleep and be ready and rested.

You have now transformed your time of insomnia into a time of reconnecting. You created a truly special, precious time. And because it was you who brought it about, insomnia's power over you has been broken.

REHABILITATION
These exercises are for daytime use.

They familiarize you with, and rehearse the basic skills necessary to turn things around at night.

You have me heard extolling the therapeutic value of writing, journaling, morning pages, diary keeping. There is no doubt in my mind that you too would benefit if you expressed yourself for twenty minutes a day—got things out of your system. It is an article of faith for most psychotherapies that getting things out is better than keeping them in. Experiment with what happens when you write dialogue instead of narrative. Start with your doubts:

I don't know about this writing. Does it make sense to you?

You can't really know until you tried it.

I guess that's true.

I am confused by who is who and who makes whom do what.

147

I have been confused by that every time you cheat on your diet.

You have a point there.

Next in line is getting better at **letting go**.

Letting go is so important that it warrants a chapter all by itself.

HOW to let go.

> As you are reading this your phone rings.
> *Let it go*
> You are about to freshen your drink.
> *Let it go*
> You remember one more thing to do.
> *Let it go*
> You replay a possible slight at the office.
> *Let it go*

You see?

It is like flexing your hand: holding on, letting go. Take a pen: Grab it—let it go.

That's what you want to be able to do with a thought. Once you can do it with a nagging thought, you can derail predictable feelings in its wake. Eventually.

WHY letting go is a vital skill

- If you can't let go, you'll end up suffering from mental and probably also physiological constipation. The things on your mind will

eventually crowd out all room.
- If you won't let go, life, circumstances, others will take things out of your hands against your will—often by force.
- If you don't learn to let go, your circuits will overload and you'll be a candidate for *losing it* one day.
- If you can't put things down, you'll find yourself in little and big wars most of the time. When nobody lets go, you have a tug-of-war.
- If you don't know how to put things down, you'll work too much, eat too much, drink too much, talk too much, shop too much, stay on the Internet too much, worry too much, even love too much—you are *en route* to becoming addicted.
- Once you are addicted, '*letting go and letting God*' may be your last and only chance before all is taken from you.

If you are a born hunter and gatherer, letting go of anything is like taking a bone from a dog. Go easy and start small.

Here is a visual letting-go exercise that can be practiced any time you are waiting at a traffic light.

Notice how your eyes don't want to let go of fixating on that red light? You got yourself convinced that you're going to miss the green if you take your eyes off. That is not only not true, it is actually slowing down your reaction time. In martial arts this is called using *soft eyes*, and here is what you do:

Look at that billboard at about 10 o'clock or 2 o'clock

off your visual field. The object of your compulsive stare will still be visible, just not in the center of your visual field. See how long you can do that without frantic double-checking. When the light changes you'll be able to process it without that little visceral startle effect, and pull right out. You can make a game out of it. Next time at a red light, look over to your left. Notice your next-door road-companion staring at the light as well—unless he is on the phone! He is also afraid he might be missing something most important. Now, assume your soft-eye stance, and watch who starts up first. Nine times out of ten, it will be you.

Next, practice intercepting auditory compulsions. Some of the most pervasive and disturbing ones are the telephone or being paged. We all know people who simply HAVE TO answer the phone.

Let it roll over to your answering service.

Do that three times a day.

Do you know under what circumstances you tend to lose perspective and become close minded? Do you know what subjects and issues get you "hard eyed" every time? If you don't, those next to you will definitely know. Ask them.

Make a list of these topics. Share it and get it as comprehensive as possible. Name or number your "issues." Now you can call them, and own them before they own you.

Now learn some letting-go lines that come in handy in conversations that usually drag you into compulsory involvement:

I WANT TO SLEEP

The classic *Mmhm ... yes, I can see that...*
You thought long and hard about that, didn't you?
That surely is a different perspective!
That's fascinating, how ever did you think of that?
Then what happened?
I can only imagine...
This is really important to you.
Could we get back to that tomorrow?

You remain present, but you don't engage and pick up.

You are practicing letting go so you know how to switch to "soft eyes" when nightly obsessions are about to take over.

Right now, if you will, write down an emotional hurt. Fold the paper, and hold it in your hand and in your mind. See it in your mind's eye. Feel the burn in your gut. As you are slowly putting it down on your desk, you know that it will have to stay there until you intentionally pick it back up, unfold it, and reread it. While it is folded up on your desk you are not thinking about it. If you find yourself mentally going back to it—pick up the paper as well, unfold it and read it. Then, when you feel ready to let go, put the paper down again Back-and-forth; back-and-forth.

Letting go of a thought—*for the time being*—is a glorious skill to have.

Being able to let go of a feeling is a feat for saints.

If you know anything about bipolarity, or just plain depression, you know how scarily unreliable the reality-takes of feelings alone can be. If we only could get, or

151

regain perspective, let go when we are being thrown off course by our own scare tactics. That is the purpose of "soft eyes": staying calm and centered in the face of scary stuff. "Hard eyes" throw off your breathing, tense your stomach, and increase your vulnerability.

If you are interested in practicing letting go of feelings, I suggest starting with good ones.

Why would one want to let go of a good feeling? For practice purposes; it's easier. There is less ego at stake, and you can always reclaim the feeling later again. After all this is just a training run.

> Think of a feeling as if you were holding a baby; we say that people "hold on to feelings." Get a sense for where in you body you carry it. Good feelings we often carry in our heart region. See it cradled there, cherish it, and nurse it with some breathing-And now notice how you have been kind of looking down on that feeling. You are no longer completely identified with it. You are kindly looking in on it. Now there is a difference between you and your feeling. Letting go is a process of dis-identifying. At this stage you could let it go, and focus on something else.

RESISTANCES

Even getting better can be scary, and when things get scary we tend to make excuses, slow down or drop out. Expect resistances because changing from insomnia-fighting to peace-making with yourself is scary and unsettling.

I WANT TO SLEEP

The other day around noon, while walking back to my car, I overheard one side of a conversation. A young woman, not four feet behind me, spoke loudly to a friend on her phone.

Michaela, please she said, *you gotta talk to me. I am walking here by myself and I am at least ten minutes from my dorm. I know you are with your aunt, but please? Talk to me.*

This was not a matter of security; it was the middle of the day on a busy sidewalk. It was a matter of hating to be alone. What will she do at night? How will she tolerate the minutes before unconsciousness relieves her of her own company or the lack thereof?

What if the last thing I want to do is to be alone with myself? a horrified patient asked me. *Being alone with myself is where all the trouble starts. I can't stand it!*

Extreme? I don't think so. Many people pick up the phone the minute they get home. TVs are on in all rooms literally day and night. Our days are masterworks of mental distractions. Audiovisual stimuli incessantly keep our attention riveted to outside signals. Being tuned in (to others) and responsive at all times, is what successful careers are all about. In the meantime your own inner signals are being ignored. When you are finally all alone, self-encounters are overloaded with unfinished personal business. This kind of neglect leaves you, your personal concerns, and your very own troubles unattended. Sometimes for months or even years. You are now ripe for insomnia. How about your life? Not just your daughter's? How about your happiness? Not just your customers'?

These insomnia-showdowns, as you well know, are scary and deeply unsettling. But they can also be transformed into an opportunity, heard as a plea for your attention.

Seeing insomnia in this light makes all the difference. It changes your inner climate from apprehension to reluctant appreciation. You are now in a much better frame of mind to face your next night.

When you find yourself resisting, don't just act it out. Write it out!

> *I don't have time to do try this approach because I am up against a deadline, I'll try it when I get a break and a couple of bad nights won't matter.*
> *I don't want to do these exercises because I know they won't work.*
> *I don't know enough people to start a sleep group.*

Now write: *thank you, I can appreciate your hesitations.* Then—very gently—address each of your concerns. NOT to change your mind but to keep the communication going. Sleeping comes not from doing everything right but from having a friend in yourself.

Let's end on a light note. I know insomnia is serious business, but heaviness is overrated as far as sleep is concerned. Lying awake affords a much needed opportunity to work with our mind. How about we call it 'playing' instead?

Play with your mind, instead of letting your mind play games with you?